Prai

AIDS: DON'T DIE OF PREJUDICE

"This is an immensely important and readable survey of some of the most unforgivable regimes on the planet, which, when they could so easily protect their populations from the scourge of HIV, seem to go out of their way, through wilful ignorance, prejudice, bigotry, superstition and pride, to encourage the virus to spread amongst their most vulnerable populations. The epidemic released from its first emergence a Pandora's box of social and physiological co-infections into the world, and these Norman Fowler reveals lucidly and with real passion and compassion. As with the Pandora's box of legend, there does remain a bedraggled but resolute figure of hope, banging on the box and clamouring to be released. It is impossible to read this without rising anger at such intolerance, cruelty and injustice and rising admiration at the courage, fortitude and resolution of those who try so hard to fight it."

Stephen Fry

AIDS

DON'T DIE OF PREJUDICE

NORMAN FOWLER

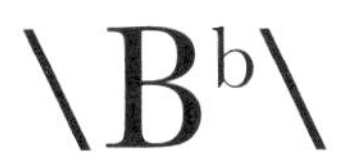

First published in Great Britain in 2014 by
Biteback Publishing Ltd
Westminster Tower
3 Albert Embankment
London SE1 7SP

ISBN 978-1-84954-704-8

10 9 8 7 6 5 4 3 2 1

A CIP catalogue record for this book is available from the British Library.

Set in Charter by Soapbox

Printed and bound in Great Britain by
CPI Group (UK) Ltd, Croydon CR0 4YY

In memory of
Tony Newton and Donald Acheson

CONTENTS

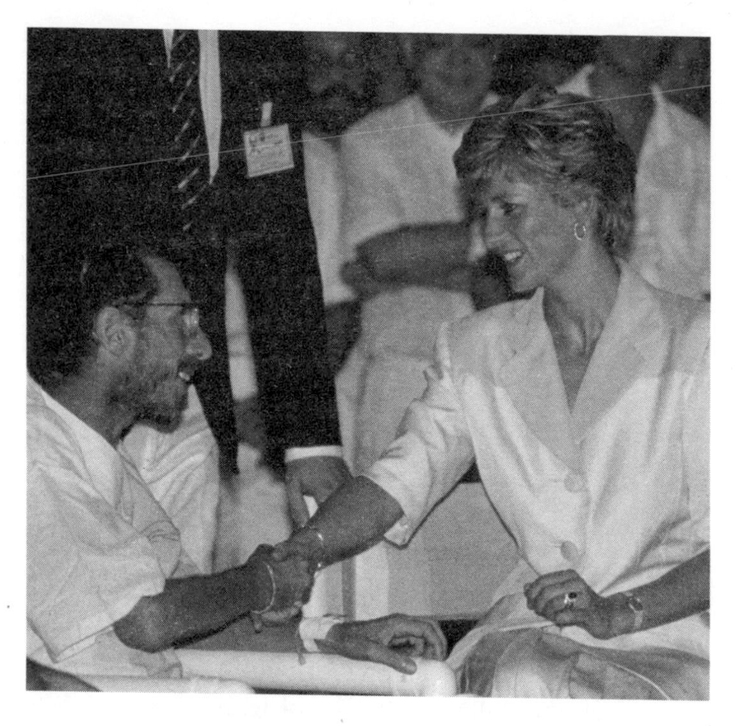

'HIV does not make people dangerous to know.'
Princess Diana, 1987.

INTRODUCTION

THE CHALLENGE

WHY IS THIS book called *Don't Die of Prejudice*? Almost thirty years ago I ran a campaign in Britain warning of the dangers of Aids called 'Don't Die of Ignorance'. It was at a time when our knowledge was limited and there were no drugs that could be used to combat HIV, the cause of Aids. It was a death sentence. Young men and women filled the hospital wards around the world but there was nothing that the doctors and nurses – themselves working under enormous strain – could do to avert the developing tragedy. It was vital that the public were warned of the danger we faced. We needed to understand.

Today, much has changed. In particular, we now have drugs that can preserve life. Yet, in spite of the medical advances, there remains the scandal of over 2 million new infections a year and over 1.5 million deaths. Over thirty-five million people worldwide live with HIV. Ignorance of how to prevent HIV is still vast and in the absence of public education campaigns it has increased over the last twenty years.

Worst of all, today millions of men and women who are already infected do not know their condition – and continue to spread the virus to others. They have not been tested, let alone treated. They may live in countries with undeveloped health systems; they may face long journeys to their nearest hospitals; or, worst of all, they may be the victims of prejudice, discrimination and stigma. Governments have made homosexuality a criminal offence in seventy-eight countries around the world. But that is a too convenient, blanket excuse.

All too often such laws are not condemned but supported by the public in those countries. The reaction of families and communities to any evidence that a person is gay or lesbian or is the victim of HIV is a huge deterrent to testing. The penalty for disclosure in many parts of the world is to be thrown out of the family home and out of work. Similar discrimination against sex workers, drug users and transgender people only adds to the tragedy. This prejudice encourages secrecy and facilitates the spread of HIV- and Aids-related deaths around the world.

MY INVOLVEMENT IN Aids began as the pandemic began to unfold. Between 1981 and 1987 I was Secretary of State for Health in Margaret Thatcher's government, and Chapter One of this book looks back at what we did then, and the obstacles we faced. After leaving government I kept in touch with the progress of the efforts to halt the spread of HIV and Aids. I worked with voluntary organisations like the Terrence Higgins Trust and in 2011 headed a House of Lords Select Committee on HIV/Aids which examined the position in Britain (which I will return to in Chapter Ten). I remain Vice-Chairman of the All-Party Parliamentary Group on HIV and Aids and am currently also on the board of the International Aids Vaccine Initiative and the patron of the British HIV Association.

I do not claim that this short book covers every nation in the world or every issue. It is not an official report or an academic treatise. My intention is instead to report on some of the most important and urgent issues that nations are facing today. It is based upon visits to nine cities of the world between November 2012 and February 2014, ranging from the Cold War capitals of Moscow and Washington to the cities of the future like Cape Town and New Delhi. The undiagnosed certainly propel the figures in Africa and Asia but they do also in the United States and Europe. For once, we all face an issue – which cannot be ignored on the basis that it is 'over there' or 'out of sight' in some distant land.

We now have antiretroviral drugs and the promise they give to patients of a full and active life. The prices have come down, cheaper generics have been introduced and all the patient has to do now is take one or two tablets a day rather than the cocktail of twenty drugs or more required a few years ago.

As far as drug users are concerned, the clean-needles policy has been proved effective and has been emulated by a range of countries. The trusty condom continues to show its worth in spite of some damaging attacks by people who must have known better, and male circumcision has been proven as a valuable means of preventing disease. We might not have a vaccine or a cure, but we have the means to at least contain the virus – and yet the casualties continue to build up not just in their thousands but in their millions.

That is why for this book I wanted to find out more about what is happening, not only in Britain but in other countries around the world. For HIV and Aids is self-evidently an international epidemic in which around thirty-six million men, women and children have so far perished – yes, *thirty-six million*. The drugs which will preserve life are now available, but still we have over 1,600,000 deaths a year. Surely we can do better than that? Surely there is a duty on us to preserve the lives that are being so squandered?

In the 1980s we had the excuse that we did not have the drugs to prevent death – but what is the excuse today? There is no doubt about what has shocked me most on my travels. In a word, it is prejudice: the official and personal prejudice against minorities which stands today as a massive barrier to public health throughout the world.

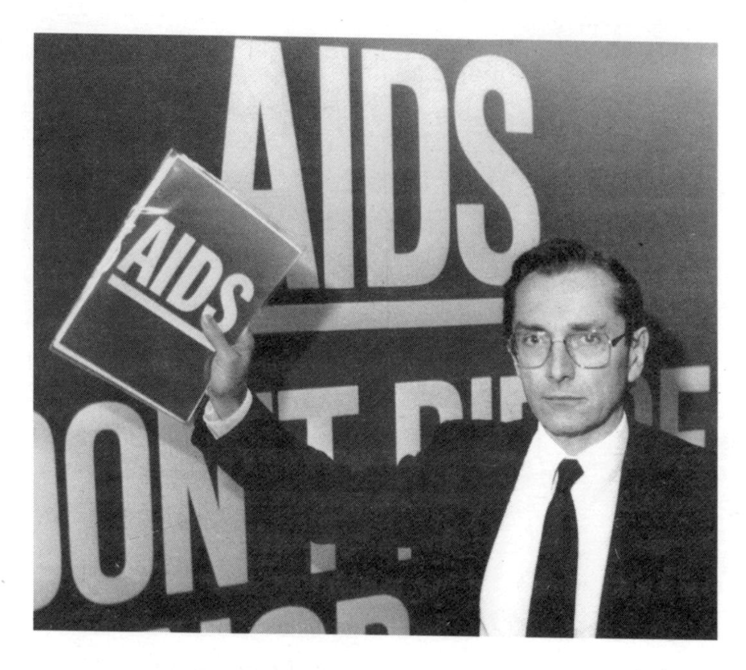

Norman Fowler launching the 'Don't Die of Ignorance' campaign, 1986.

ONE

AIDS AND THE IRON LADY

I CANNOT REMEMBER with any clarity the first time that the Aids issue came onto my desk. I can remember much more exactly the time I became seriously frustrated about the way we in Margaret Thatcher's government were handling the crisis. It was almost thirty years ago and I was Health and Social Security Secretary in her Cabinet. By the beginning of 1986, Aids cases were beginning to increase alarmingly. We were struggling to explain to the public the danger they faced and also to persuade other ministers that urgent measures were now needed. My view was that we needed a direct advertising campaign explaining how the virus was contracted and warning that there were no drugs or vaccinations that could be used to counter it. The prospect for those who ignored these warnings was death. It was that which justified (or so I thought) the government going into detail on sexual practices and drug taking – information that was a million miles away from the usual advertising emanating from Whitehall. It was not a time to be too delicate. People needed to understand and to protect themselves, but this approach landed me in immediate and potentially fatal trouble. Standing in the way of such a blunt approach was the Iron Lady herself.

Our aim was to mount a newspaper advertising campaign in the early part of 1986. In February I circulated a draft advertisement to all the ministers represented on the General Home Affairs Committee of the Cabinet ('H') which took the major decisions on domestic policy. I also sent it to Margaret Thatcher's office at 10 Downing Street. I warned that of the 275 cases of Aids reported by the end of 1985, 144 had died. My warning was that, on present trends, there would be over 20,000 people, mostly men, infected with the HIV virus by 1988. Most would be unaware of their condition and would continue to spread the infection. In an attempt to smooth the way past ministers, I explained that the warning advertisements would have to 'strike a balance between being too explicit and too anodyne'.

That explanation did not carry the Prime Minister. On the morning set for the 'H' committee meeting, we received a phone call from Margaret Thatcher's office. She had read my paper and had responded with a terse comment. 'Do we have to have the section on risky sex?' she asked. 'I should have thought that it could do immense harm if teenagers read it.' Her fear was that young people would in some way be contaminated by this knowledge. The 'risky sex' section of which the Prime Minister was complaining started with a warning on the dangers of sexual intercourse with an infected person and repeated what was to become our familiar message on the importance of using a condom. It went on: 'Anal (back passage) intercourse involves the highest risk and should be avoided. Obviously any act that damages the penis, vagina, anus or mouth is dangerous, particularly if it causes bleeding. Even wet kissing with an infected person may be risky.'

It brought us up against some of the basic questions concerned with any public education campaign on Aids. Were we to muffle our message so that the chance of causing offence was minimised? Did we really believe as a government that by describing hitherto unknown sexual practices we encouraged innocent young people to follow suit? Or did we take the view that these fears were fanciful and that unless we did describe what we were talking about we would fail in our task? Although these questions may seem dated, they raise some of the same issues that stand in the way of a sensible policy on sex education in British schools to this day. To do justice to the ministers on 'H' committee back in 1986 (and in spite of the attempted steer from No. 10), they not only approved the draft advertisement but asked me to look at extending the campaign to other media. Willie Whitelaw, the chairman of the committee and leader of the House of Lords, summed up, albeit with a nod to Mrs T., that 'the committee agreed that the campaign should proceed as planned and thought that the explicit references to sexual practices were a regrettable necessity'.

The advertisement, which, frankly, was hardly earth-shattering, limped towards publication – but not before Margaret Thatcher had launched one further depth-charge. A week after the committee had agreed to the text, my office received a letter from her principal private secretary, Nigel Wicks. There was no beating about the bush.

> *The Prime Minister has emphasised that she still remains against certain parts of the advertisement. She thinks that the anxiety on the part of parents and many teenagers, who would never be in danger from Aids, would exceed the good which the advertisement might do. In her view it would be better to follow the 'VD' precedent of putting notices in doctors' surgeries, public lavatories etc. But to place advertisements in newspapers which every young person could read and learn of practices they never knew about would, in her view, do harm.*

These, I was told, were the Prime Minister's 'firmly held views' and that now I might 'wish to consider showing the Prime Minister an amended advertisement which omits the parts which, in the Prime Minister's view, would be likely to offend'. History had, in fact, already proven the efficacy of blunt sexual health advice. There had been public health campaigns about sex long before we went into this apparently forbidden territory. In both the First World War and the Second there had been campaigns which had warned against venereal disease and which had resulted in no known harm to young people. In the 1939–45 conflict, the chief medical officer actually went on BBC radio to warn the public – young and old – of the dangers. All the evidence was that the campaigns had reduced sexually transmitted disease. As for the Prime Minister's idea of confining messages to public lavatories and surgeries, there was no evidence that in the late 1980s, with all modern communication techniques at our disposal, this was remotely the best we could do. The world had moved on.

The unaltered newspaper advertisements went ahead in March and April of 1986 without much comment. We received very few complaints and there were no instances of readers burning *The Times* or *Daily Mail* in protest. My concerns about the campaign were very different from those of the Prime Minister. It had taken weeks to get to publication, even though the whole point of what we were saying was that this was an emergency. Nor was I convinced that closely written text – rather like the instructions on a medicine bottle – delivered the goods. It was an inauspicious start to what was to become the biggest public education campaign ever staged in Britain.

In June I circulated the draft of a new, shorter and simpler newspaper advertisement, which repeated the risky sex message of the first advertisement. It warned 'the more partners – especially male partners – someone has, the more likely it is that they will have sex with an infected person'. The sharp-eyed would also have noticed an attitude to drug taking which was appreciably softer than the conventional warning that 'drugs are wrong and we will prosecute you'. The advertisement said: 'For those who cannot give up, it is very important not to share needles or other equipment. Injecting just once with a needle that carries the virus could mean catching Aids. Best of all, don't inject.'

However, it was not the difference in tone that was picked up when the draft of this advertisement was sent around to ministers. This time the objection came from the undoubted Grand Old Man of the Thatcher government, Quintin Hailsham, the Lord Chancellor. A wayward but brilliant man who could easily have been Prime Minister, he objected not so much to the message as such but to the language being proposed. His objection was to the phrase 'having sex'. He wrote:

> *I am convinced that there must be some limit to vulgarity and illiteracy. 'Sex' means that you are either male or female. It does not mean the same thing as sexual practice. Nor does 'having sex' mean anything at all. Could they not use the literate 'sexual intercourse'? If that is thought to be too narrow then why not 'sexual relations' or 'physical sexual practices', but not 'sex' or still worse 'having sex'!!!*

Grammatically, the Lord Chancellor could not be faulted. The phrase was changed (only to reappear later on) and eventually, in July 1986, the second series of newspaper advertisements was published. It had modest success but did not match the increasing public concern that there was on the spread of Aids. We did not lack advice on what we should do.

Donald Acheson, the chief medical officer, who, with the Health Minister Tony Newton, gave me invaluable support throughout these fraught months, sent me a note on what had happened in the First World War. At one stage the British had distributed a leaflet to troops going on leave in Paris in an attempt to reduce the incidence of sexually transmitted disease. The leaflet said: 'In this new experience you may find temptations both in wine and women. You must entirely resist both temptations and while treating all women with perfect courtesy you should avoid any intimacy. Do your duty, fear God, honour the King.'

This message was less than successful. A fifth of 5,000 troops on leave in Paris became infected. The later approach was to issue prophylactic packs containing calomel ointment, and treatment rooms were set up for soldiers where they could receive urethal irrigation within twenty-four hours of exposure. Subsequently, 300,000 troops visited Paris and only 3 per cent were infected.

Yet, over half a century later, Margaret Thatcher had undoubted supporters for her untypically 'softly, softly' approach. The party chairman, Norman Tebbit, was a sceptic about whether the government should be seen to raise the profile of an issue which he judged was treated with distaste by many in middle England. As for middle Scotland, the former Scottish Secretary, George Younger, was a consistent doubter, particularly when it came to drug users, as too was the Scottish Health Minister John Mackay. And with a dominating leader like Margaret Thatcher there were always going to be ministers who would fall into line behind her on virtually any subject.

Some columnists and writers who were strong Thatcher supporters went further. Woodrow Wyatt, who had started life as a Labour MP and ended to the right of most Conservatives, left his *News of the World* readers in no doubt about his views: 'The start of Aids was homosexual love making. Promiscuous women are vulnerable, making love to promiscuous bisexuals. They then pass Aids on to normal men.' He added, 'Labour councils give grants to homosexual centres. They encourage children to experiment with sex. This is murder.' Sir Alfred Sherman, who was a close supporter of the Prime Minister and another émigré from the left, wrote to *The Times* saying that Aids was a problem of undesirable minorities: 'mainly sodomites and drug abusers together with numbers of women who voluntarily associate with the sexual underworld'.

Another writer who received attention was Christopher (now Lord) Monckton. In 1987, he wrote an article for the *American Spectator* entitled 'A British View', where he argued that 'there is only one way to stop Aids. That is to screen the entire population regularly and to quarantine all carriers of the disease for life.' He was supported by the Conservative Family Group, which proposed that people with Aids should be put into isolation units.

The most consistent attack, however, was that we were wrong to treat Aids as essentially a public health issue. Above all, our critics said, it was a moral issue. It was useless for me to reply that we were not ignoring these issues. From the beginning I had said that sticking to one faithful partner was the best advice we could give, but this was never enough for some religious leaders. An outspoken example was the then Chief Rabbi, Sir Immanuel Jakobovits, whose views on Aids were practically identical to those of Margaret Thatcher. Later in the campaign we met and he handed me an aide-memoire which, in passing, praised the 'urgency, boldness and effectiveness' of the campaign but then set out in dramatic language a view which was held by many of the so-called moral majority. Among his dozen objections to the advertising campaign, the Chief Rabbi's aide-memoire said:

> *Campaign breeds false sense of security, not to mention false values. In effect encourages promiscuity by advertising it. Introduces to many children and decent young people ideas of sex outside marriage entirely unknown to them.*

Tells people not what is right but how to do wrong and get away with it – like sending people into contaminated atmosphere but providing them with gas masks and protective clothing, or instructing thieves how to escape being caught.

The aide-memoire ended: 'Say plainly: Aids consequence of marital infidelity, premarital adventures, sexual deviation, and social irresponsibility – putting pleasure before duty and discipline.'

It was stirring stuff but it went smack against all experience. Two world wars had shown that practical advice (together with protection) was the best way of combating sexual disease. We would lack credibility with the people we wanted to influence if we were thought to be preaching. Our internal research showed that among the people we needed to convince were gay men, who took an almost cavalier attitude to the disease, and drug users, who could be apathetic to their fate. Moreover, many heterosexuals regarded Aids as not relevant to them, in spite of the advice of the chief medical officer that the potential for its spread in the heterosexual community was real. Generally, men and women – gay and straight – became more and more concerned as they read in the press or saw on television stories about the advance of Aids. They too wanted to know the medical facts as we knew them at that time. It all argued for a single campaign of education. In the words of our research document: 'There is a need for a clear accurate statement of what behaviour will lead to transmission.'

There was of course another entirely practical reason why it needed to remain a public health message. An attempt at the kind of moral message that the Chief Rabbi wanted would have been exploded instantly by the first minister revealed to be having an extramarital affair. Later, we learnt that in spades with John Major's 'back to basics' campaign in the 1990s, which was wrongly interpreted as calling for some kind of moral regeneration. My view was – and remains – that governments have authority when they put scientific or medical facts before the public, backed by the best experts at their disposal. They certainly should not undermine the churches, but they are entitled to expect that the churches themselves will continue to preach their messages on the importance of family and marriage. They never had a better opportunity than in the first years of the Aids crisis.

In the main, our course was accepted by the media. Television and radio, both independent and the BBC, ran their own programmes, and in the early days their reports were more effective than our publicity. As for the press, you paid your money and took your choice. Some newspapers pressed us to do more, others suspected we were doing too much. There was also a contrast between what the broadcasting organisations and the newspapers felt was possible for them to do. Both George Thomson, the head of the Independent Broadcasting Authority, and

Alasdair Milne, the Director General of the BBC, instantly offered me support when I went to see them. Richard Marsh, the chairman of the Newspaper Publishers Association, whom I later joined in the House of Lords, was less forthcoming. He said that usually it was as much as newspapers could do to agree on the time of day but on one point they did speak with a united voice – they never gave free advertising.

As for the public generally, the criminal law forbidding homosexuality may have been scrapped in 1967 but that had not altered attitudes overnight. Many people treated the idea of gay sex with hostility and distaste, and thought that the victims of Aids should be left to their fate. In particular, they could not understand why the government insisted on putting out a general message on Aids addressed to all when everybody knew that it was just 'a gay disease'. The accusation was that we were simply pandering to the 'gay lobby' when there was next to no chance of HIV being contracted by 'normal' heterosexual men sleeping around. Today, there are as many new cases of HIV in the United Kingdom coming from heterosexual sex as from men having sex with men.

For me it was decision time. How far was I prepared to push this campaign? Although I knew little about the gay community and at that stage had few gay friends, one reaction made me increasingly angry. I could not understand (and still don't) why there was this opposition to gays and lesbians purely on grounds of their sexual orientation. I suppose I came from the 1960s generation, whose motto, in the main, was 'live and let live'. But my major objection was the rank injustice of it. Why should they be treated as second-class citizens? I saw Aids as an issue quite apart from the usual run of health issues, like waiting lists and health service funding, which I dealt with daily. My critics said it became an obsession and perhaps it did. People were dying and my concern was that artificial barriers and prejudice should not stand in the way of doing all we could to prevent the spread of HIV.

At the Department of Health we determined to move on from our rather innocuous newspaper advertising of early 1986 to something infinitely more direct. Our next plan of action was to send leaflets explaining Aids to all 23 million households in the country. (That leaflet is included at the end of this book and still serves as an introduction to some of the basic issues of Aids.) A leaflet drop of this kind had never been attempted before with a public health campaign, and I was under no illusion about the difficulties of getting the proposal through the creaking government machine.

You did not need much imagination to forecast the objections. Would it not come smack up against Margaret Thatcher's concern that we would be teaching young people all kinds of things that they never knew before? After all, when the leaflet went through the letterbox, anyone in the household could read it. As for the language, there was a massive opportunity for objection. The words had to be direct for otherwise we would run into criticism that we were pulling our punches. On the other hand, if the words were too direct and the descriptions of sexual acts too detailed, then we would be attacked from the opposite direction. In August 1986 I wrote to 'H' committee ministers with the proposed text of the leaflet, and my fears quickly proved only too correct.

Quintin Hailsham replied that the more he reflected on my leaflet the more doubtful he became of the wisdom of proceeding. 'The appearance on every doormat of the document in question is liable to cause controversy and even offence and might well spread panic.'

From Scotland John Mackay, the Health Minister, replied: 'We run the risk of being heavily criticised both for delivering sexually explicit leaflets to every household in the country whether the occupiers wish to receive this or not and for the inadequacy of the guidance in the leaflet.'

From the Treasury, Peter Brooke, the Minister of State, urged a proper evaluation to ensure that the cost could be justified. The cost was a few million. Inevitably, he added: 'There could, of course, be no question of additional funding.'

Against these three senior ministers, the Home Secretary Douglas Hurd, the Northern Ireland Secretary Tom King and the Education Secretary Ken Baker supported the communication attempt. Hurd used words with which I totally agreed. 'We must not put ourselves in the position of having neglected our duty when that duty was clear.'

Nevertheless 'H' committee was split and Margaret Thatcher left little doubt where her sympathies lay. Her private secretary at No. 10 wrote to ministers: 'The Prime Minister is concerned that there are various risks attached to the proposal.' She proposed instead a new full-scale meeting of 'H' committee with a full draft text, together with professional advice on the likely impact. It all meant further delay and brought us to a crunch point in the campaign. It was obvious that the government machine as it stood was not up to the task of rapid response. Speedy action was impossible and all the time the position was deteriorating.

Among my team at the Health Department there was increasing frustration but there emerged also the genesis of a solution. Rather than a general committee, we thought, why not have a special Aids Cabinet committee with ministers thoroughly briefed on the position and capable of making quick decisions which could be then translated into action? There was, however, one problem. Separate Cabinet committees of this kind would most likely be chaired by Margaret Thatcher herself and be held at No. 10. Given her views, this did not seem a massively good idea. Any Cabinet minister knew what would happen. We had all experienced the Thatcher treatment. Speaking personally, it had taken me several months to get my proposals on social security reform past her. I knew exactly what would happen on Aids. The Prime Minister would ask for changes and, worst of all, reports that would need to be presented at the next meeting, which would make quick decisions – and action – impossible. The obvious solution was to have another chairman. As I was taught in my army days, 'if you come up against an immoveable object, try to go around it'.

It was at this point that two of the most skilled civil service warriors in Whitehall took a decisive hand. The first was Sir Robert Armstrong, the Cabinet Secretary and head of the civil service; the second was Sir Kenneth Stowe, who once had been the principal private secretary to the Labour Prime Minister Jim Callaghan and was now my Permanent Secretary in the department. Armstrong was entirely convinced of the seriousness of the issue and it was he who persuaded Margaret Thatcher that she had neither the time nor the need to chair this specialist committee, and that this could be done by her deputy, Willie Whitelaw, the leader of the Lords.

In the Thatcher government Whitelaw was the man everybody went to in times of trouble. He had unrivalled experience as both a former Chief Whip and Home Secretary, and was the irreplaceable number two to Margaret Thatcher herself. What no one seemed to know was that sexual health was not an entirely new area for him. Nick Edwards, the Welsh Secretary (now Lord Crickhowell), remembers that at one stage in his army service during the war Whitelaw had had oversight of sexual services for the forces in Cairo. In those days there was no debate about the message to be given: it was about proper precautions, not moral advice

– and non-observance brought in the full might of military discipline. As it happened, most of the men around the table at our special Cabinet committee had done at least some military service, which perhaps explains in part their pragmatic attitude. I certainly remember being marched in as a young national serviceman to watch a public information film on sexual disease which made my efforts seem rather like the vicar's monthly newsletter.

As might be imagined, Whitelaw treated Aids very much as the old soldier might. He was not going to make moral judgements. He wanted to see the public protected and he wanted to make progress. It was an inspired appointment from my point of view. The committee was set up with some of the most powerful members of the Cabinet on it, but without either Quintin Hailsham or Norman Tebbit. We met for the first time on Tuesday 11 November 1986 in the large ministerial conference room in the bowels of the House of Commons. The change was almost instantaneous. Proposals that were blocked – like the Aids leaflet – suddenly became unblocked. The committee shared ownership. Rather than a prevaricating response of 'I am not sure about that' the reaction became 'we must make progress'.

In less than two months we took a series of decisions which entirely transformed the government's position. The leaflet for the letterbox drop was approved without opposition, and their delivery, and an accompanying media campaign, was planned for January 1987.

The only flak came from outside government. At a party meeting in Manchester I was told by one questioner that I was simply encouraging safe promiscuity and by another that she would burn any leaflet that came to her house to keep it away from her fifteen-year-old daughter. Then, in an intervention which lacked all compassion, James Anderton, the then chief constable of Manchester, used a training seminar in December 1986 to accuse homosexuals, drug addicts and prostitutes who had Aids 'of swirling in a cess pit of their own making'. At a conference in Scarborough of the Young Conservatives, one speaker received what sounded like thunderous applause for echoing Anderton's views. The noise from Anderton's supporters may have been great but, when it came to the vote, the motion backing the government's position was passed overwhelmingly. It confirmed my view that the public thought the matter was too serious for fake remedies and were on our side.

There is an intriguing postscript on Anderton which resulted from the publication in early 2014 of declassified government papers from 1986. The *Manchester Evening News* discovered that Margaret Thatcher had come to his support when it was proposed that to avoid fresh disasters he should set out his future speaking engagements. Margaret Thatcher's private secretary wrote to the Home Office saying: 'The Prime Minister has commented that it would be outrageous if the chief constable were required to seek clearance for all his public speaking engagements.' At a meeting with Home Office officials, Anderton said that he was 'governed in all that he did by his religious beliefs and that indeed police officers were daily called upon in court to take an oath on the Bible. Religious beliefs and police work could not therefore be entirely separated.'

On another issue the Aids Cabinet committee was split: how to deal with injecting drug users. My diary takes up the story:

> Wednesday 3 December 1986. *The fifth meeting of the Aids committee. The main issue is drugs. Should we give free needles to drug injectors so that at least they have clean needles rather than share them and spread the virus? My case is that this is one of the chief ways in which the disease spreads – particularly into the heterosexual population. I see the difficulties – encouraging drug misuse etc – but believe that provided such schemes are controlled then we should go ahead. I am not advocating free needles in every shop! Clean needles should be part of a series of measures aimed at reducing drug misuse and that therefore means counselling. Douglas Hurd supports me but Malcolm Rifkind – who has the worst problem of all in Scotland – is very sceptical. Can we be sure it will do good? If it goes ahead it must be monitored. George Younger is totally opposed. He simply does not believe it can be right to recognise in this way an illegal activity. The*

other members of the committee are sceptical. In situations like this the position of the chairman is vital. On the views expressed Willie Whitelaw would have been quite entitled to have ruled that the proposals were rejected. Instead he asked me to work up proposals for pilot schemes which we would consider later in the month. Willie is entirely invaluable.

In those months back in late 1986 and the beginning of 1987, it was the opposition of the Scottish Office to the policy of clean needles which was the most difficult to overcome – and also the most difficult to understand. In the autumn of 1986 an expert committee actually set up by the Scottish Health Department had reported that HIV infection among intravenous drug users was higher in Scotland than in the rest of the United Kingdom. The committee found there was a particular problem in Edinburgh, where the police confiscated syringes and needles from anyone found in possession of them, and this had resulted in widespread sharing of equipment. There was no doubt about their recommendation.

It is of the utmost importance that those who continue to inject are persuaded to use clean equipment and never share it. Clean equipment should therefore not be denied to those who cannot be dissuaded from injection ... On balance the prevention of the spread should take priority over any perceived risk of increased drug misuse.

The committee found that there was also a prevailing medical opposition to maintenance prescribing, even though this had a double benefit in that it usually meant prescribing methadone, which not only is taken orally but also brought the user into contact with drug services. None of this persuaded Scottish ministers, and it was only when Michael Forsyth became health minister after the June 1987 election that the policy of clean needles and methadone was conclusively endorsed.

Almost a month after our December meeting on drug use I ran into fresh opposition from No. 10. I had proposed that there should be a ministerial broadcast to warn of the dangers of Aids but this was not at all the Iron Lady's view. My diary again takes up the story:

> Tuesday 30 December 1986. *Christmas comes to an end ... Willie Whitelaw and the Aids committee had approved our plan to have a ministerial broadcast on Aids. Late in the afternoon the news comes through that the Prime Minister has vetoed the idea. She hasn't had a ministerial broadcast on any subject over the last seven years and does not intend to start now with Aids. She believes it would give an impression of panic and crisis. It is a great pity that we didn't know this before as we already have a crew lined up to produce it and I have approached Michael Meacher [the shadow Health Minister] on the basis that this is not party political controversial. He has agreed that Labour*

don't want a right of reply. My main fear is that the story of the change will leak and the whole campaign will be dented on the basis that Margaret is distancing herself from it.

Wednesday 31 December 1986. *My view is that we are both missing an opportunity and also running the risk of a leak by cancelling our plan for the broadcast. I get Nigel Wicks to ring me. He is at his most bureaucratic and says that it is in the notes of procedure that the Prime Minister must be consulted before any official approach is made: the consent of a Cabinet committee is not enough. I growl at him that we are rather past that point now and that unless we are careful we will be embroiled in a public row on the cancellation. Wicks obviously feels 'and whose fault is that?' – but is tactful enough not to say so. He suggests more constructively that the best approach to the PM is by pointing out that the ministerial broadcast is a public health message and not just a minister speaking straight to camera. I say the issue is urgent and I better see her as soon as possible. Back comes the message an hour later – come to No. 10 at 7.00 p.m.*

It is a curious way of celebrating New Year's Eve but I go to No. 10 and up to her study where she offers me a whisky. She says that she is not doing anything in the evening – 'too much work to be done'. It becomes clear after one minute flat that she will not be changed on the ministerial broadcast. She says that she has not had one on the Falklands, on the riots or on any other health issue. She thinks I will get quite enough publicity from news broadcasts and it is more effective. On some issues it is worth having an argument but this is not one of them. There is no prospect of her changing her mind. I hate to admit it but we would have saved ourselves a lot of trouble had we found this out before. This part over we then talked more widely. She was at her best – relaxed, intelligent, sympathetic. She has difficulties in her attitude to Aids. She recognises it as a profoundly serious health threat but another part of her would like to see us putting all our efforts into reducing waiting lists or giving further help in other disease areas. At one point she says to me: 'You mustn't become known as just the minister for Aids.' Her (kind) point was that my party conference speech had gone exceptionally well and there were other frontiers in politics. True as this may be I think I have a duty (if that doesn't sound too pompous) to inform the public of the dangers. My fear would be that unless we do this then in five years' time the judgement will be that the government 'didn't do enough'. I do not believe that can be said now but we must ensure that it remains the case.

As it happened we were not pursued by the press on the 'U-turn' over the broadcast, which was just as well. I saw much later the guidance given to our press officers. The only answer they were to give if journalists asked why the broadcast had been cancelled was: 'It was a government decision'; if they were asked whether Margaret Thatcher had vetoed the idea, their only instruction was: 'Do not be drawn further.'

In January 1987, as the leaflets arrived in households throughout the country, our campaign went even more high profile. Posters had been going up on billboards up and down the country, proclaiming 'AIDS. DON'T DIE OF IGNORANCE' accompanied by the message: 'Gay or Straight. Male or Female. Anyone can get Aids from sexual intercourse. So the more partners, the greater the risk. Protect yourself. Use a condom.' To accompany the leaflet-drop, we commissioned a television campaign. Before Christmas, the advertising agency TBWA had showed us what they had come up with, but as I wrote in my diary 'they were too reminiscent of trailers for a horror film – Apocalypse Three'. Changes were made and what went on screen were the now-famous 'tombstone' ads. A drill cut out the word 'Aids' on a slab of rock: the sepulchral voiceover of John Hurt warned: 'There is now a danger that has become a threat to us all. It is a deadly disease and there is no known cure.' The advertisement ended with a bunch of white lilies on top of the gravestone and the picture of our leaflet. 'Read this leaflet when it arrives. If you ignore Aids it could be the death of you.' We followed this up with an advertisement showing the present problem as the tip of the iceberg: 'Unless we act now it's going to get much, much worse.' As these appeared on both TV channels, the agency ran campaigns for cinema and radio. The campaign was inevitably criticised by some as being over the top and altogether too Hollywood. My reply is that, in all the comments that have been made to me over the years that followed, there is no doubt that it was the television advertisements which had most impact and did most to save lives.

Throughout our campaign I sought lessons from abroad. My view has always been that this was one of the best ways of getting a perspective on the problems we face in Britain. In my period in government I was surprised how little this was done. 'The Foreign Office is there for "diplomacy",' I wrote in my diary at the time. 'We have them now thinking commercially but not yet on social policy.' I travelled to the World Health Organization in Geneva where Jonathan Mann, the founder and first director of the WHO's Global Program on Aids (who died tragically early in a 1998 air crash) told me that in his estimate there would be between 500,000 and 3 million deaths over the next five years. One of the warnings he gave was against 'sex tourism' where men from the developed world travelled to the Third World with the promise of sexual partners, male or female, to be provided. I went to Berlin with its dividing wall and its eerie, flood-lit no man's land between East and West. There, a gay rights organisation complimented us on our campaign (to the amazement of at least one British journalist there) and hoped the German government would follow suit. In my diary I wrote:

> *My lasting impression, however, is of a consultant in charge of sexually transmitted disease at the main Berlin hospital. A gaunt man he was obviously working under very considerable strain. He thought the position was already bad and was quite likely to become disastrous. He had lost twelve patients over the last two weeks – predominantly young men. In our emphasis on prevention we must never forget the compassion that is needed for those who are dying – or the support that is needed for the staff working with Aids sufferers.*

In Amsterdam I saw in action the 'methadone bus' which went direct to drug users and exchanged dirty needles for clean ones. 'It seems to work well here,' I wrote, 'but that does not necessarily mean that it will work well in Edinburgh.' Then, early in January 1987, I left for the United States to seek guidance from their experience, given that they had a much greater problem than we in Britain. My hopes were high that this usually imaginative and innovative nation would have further answers. I was disappointed. My diary gives a glimpse of how the epidemic was being handled then across the Atlantic.

San Francisco

Sunday 18 January 1987. *San Francisco has by any standards a major Aids crisis. The city – probably the most beautiful in the United States – became a centre for the gay population during the 1960s and '70s. The consul general says 'they became respectable'. They never were accepted, of course, by everybody and Aids has led not only to a backlash against them but confirmed the opposition of those who were always reluctant to accept them in the first place. Many of the health workers here compliment me as a minister taking a lead. This was seen as being in contrast to their position. Nobody can remember President Reagan ever having said anything about Aids.*

Tuesday 20 January 1987. *Press and television interest hits a new high. It is not something we have sought. Indeed my fear was that they would interrupt the briefing sessions. In fact they have not intruded and if some of the messages we are receiving are transmitted back home then that would be very positive health education. The scale of the problem is coming through to the reporters and not all of them enjoy covering the subject. There is at least one writer who has asked his office not to put him on Aids again. But without fail the press and television party are taking the visit seriously and are not attempting to score points.*

Inevitably the point of attention for the media is my visit to San Francisco general hospital – an early twentieth-century complex of red-brick buildings on what was once the edge of the city. I talk to the nurses who are working under stress but with enormous commitment. The girl who has worked there longest – almost three years – is obviously going through something of a crisis herself. She has seen her patients die without being able to do anything to intervene. We will see what she does. My guess is that in spite of all the difficulties she will stay. On average staff stay longer in the Aids unit than other parts of the hospital. I then went into the patient ward. One of the patients had agreed to be televised and photographed as we shook hands. He was a young man in his thirties – the average age in San Francisco for Aids cases. He was remarkably cheerful and anxious to talk. He had been a shipping clerk but now there was no prospect of him working, although his employer would have been happy for him to come in for an hour or so a day. We talked for a few minutes. I was photographed shaking hands and I left to continue the tour. He was a brave man who would be dead in the next two or three months.

Washington

Thursday 22 January 1987. *We stay the night at the residence in Washington and Anthony Acland [the British Ambassador to Washington], a rather aloof withdrawn man, welcomes us. I do not get the impression that Aids is top of his list of interests and I suppose inevitably his mind is on American and particularly Washington politics. We have the biggest embassy of any in Washington which always strikes me as showing an exaggerated view of our international importance. I suppose my real feeling is that the Foreign Office take a rather superior view of the domestic problems of Britain and regard themselves as a cut above everybody else in Whitehall – ministers included. Overnight it has started snowing. The big Cadillac cannot make it down the drive to the residence and on the roads the traffic is slow moving. We just about make it to Bathesda to talk research at the National Institute of Health. Our talks confirm a number of impressions. In particular in spite of the unprecedented effort being made to develop a vaccine and a cure, no one is optimistic of any immediate break-through. The other message is also clear: in Britain we may be doing a great deal on public education but the Americans are devoting enormous resources to research. When we make our way back to downtown Washington the road conditions are chaotic. Our driver tells us that government departments have been sent home because of the snow. However we do manage to keep an appointment with Otis Bowen, the US Health Secretary. He is a doctor himself but now over seventy. I had met him before both in Washington and Geneva and liked him as gentle and restrained man. What, however, is clear is that neither he nor the administration intend to take a lead on public education. 'That', says Bowen, 'is a matter for local decision.'*

New York

Friday 23 January 1987. *Washington airport is shut so instead we take the Amtrak train up to New York. The problem in New York is drugs. The city health department paint a bleak picture of New York in 1987. They estimate that there are about 200,000 intravenous drug users. Some of them can be influenced not to share needles, but everybody believes that drug users are a more difficult group to influence than homosexuals. Many gays are well-educated, middle-class and certainly do not want to die from Aids. Some drug users are the same, but the fear is that many are apathetic about their prospects. A third of HIV cases are drug addicts, but the numbers are increasing. Beneath the surface there are tales of pure tragedy. So far 165 babies have been born with Aids: most have died within five years.*

Saturday 24 January 1987. *We visit the Roman Catholic run St Clare's Hospital. I speak to two women patients. One is twenty-three with a small baby; the other just over thirty with two children. They are both injecting drug users and they will both be dead in the next six months. Happily the children are not infected, but what a waste. Both women are articulate and intelligent – eminently capable of being good mothers. In both cases what will happen is that the children will be brought up by their grandparents.*

Sunday 25 January 1987. *Back at Heathrow Donald Acheson and I shake hands, although we will be seeing each other tomorrow. I think he realises that this trip has been for me both physically and emotionally gruelling.*

Monday 26 January 1987. *Back to the Department. A mountain of press cuttings on the American trip awaits me. The other ministers at the morning meeting tell me of the television coverage which they say was both massive and good. I gather this feeling is not shared at either No. 10 or Central Office. A* Daily Mail *report says that Margaret Thatcher and Norman Tebbit are 'exasperated' by the education campaign. I guess that this has come from Norman himself who over the years has used this particular Mail correspondent to report his unhelpful views. But it is too late for them to intervene now. The campaign is launched and it cannot be reversed. Frankly if they do not like it they can lump it.*

It was shortly after my return from the United States that we had one enormous fillip. I visited Middlesex Hospital, which was one of the major Aids hospitals in London. A new ward had been created. It was light and airy and was to be opened in March by Princess Diana, and there was now much press speculation about whether she would shake hands with patients, as I had done in my visit to patients in San Francisco. It was a mark of the apprehension that still prevailed, in spite of all our efforts to say that Aids could not be passed in this way. Of course Diana did shake hands and, in photographs that sped around the world, demonstrated that the fears were based on ignorance. There was never a better ambassador than the young princess.

So what were the overall results of our work? It certainly showed that the government machine was capable of swift decision-making. In a matter of a few months we had implemented a massive public education campaign, communicated directly to the public what they should do to avoid the all too likely death sentence which came from Aids, and had started a policy to help one of the most unpopular groups in Britain – injecting drug users. But, more than that, I would claim that we also demonstrated that public education campaigns can be effective. Our Aids campaign was regularly checked by attitude research carried out by Gallup. In my last weeks at the Department of Health (before I moved to the Employment Department after the June 1987 election) Gallup produced their latest report. Well over 90 per cent of the public had seen the advertising, 94 per cent thought that the government was right to be doing the advertising they had seen and only 7 per cent found some of the things 'offensive';

knowledge of what caused Aids and what did not had massively increased and condom use had increased, with a third of the sample believing that the main message was that using a condom reduced risk. There was even an answer to the Chief Rabbi, with a third taking the view that the main message was 'don't sleep around / few partners / stop permissive behaviour'.

Later research showed that, as well as a reduction in HIV, there was a marked fall in sexual disease generally. One public health analyst commenting today on the campaign said: 'Within the space of a couple of years there was a dramatic fall in gonorrhoea and syphilis. No other change could explain this drop.' Sadly this did not persuade succeeding governments to follow suit. Getting resources from the Treasury for advertising is always difficult and getting them for something as 'sensitive' as sexual disease is even more so. It can leave a government open to attack and even in my time at the Health Department there were grumbles from the inside that I had robbed other policy areas of their 'fair share'. So, rather than the campaign on Aids being properly continued and developed into sexual health generally, the message faded. No one claims that exactly the same tactics would work year after year – that is why you have advertising agencies to develop campaigns. As it was, the most successful public health campaign since the Second World War was followed by years of inaction.

In the end, the most permanently successful result was the decision to introduce clean needles. This secured a lasting reduction in the numbers of new infections by the injecting drug route. In Britain a tiny proportion of drug users – around 1 per cent – now acquire HIV through shared needles. Nor has there ever been any evidence that the policy has increased drug misuse. When I chaired a House of Lords Select Committee on HIV in 2011 I specifically asked this question of the chief constables. They had received no complaints of that kind. The initial fears had been misplaced.

And Margaret Thatcher? Over the years I have pondered on my New Year's Eve meeting at Downing Street with the Prime Minister and her remark that 'you mustn't become known as just the minister for Aids'. I fear that my diary interpretation of her words was too generous. Her words bore the obvious meaning. She meant: 'Go and do something else.' Her aim was that by use of charm and flattery she could move me on and away from Aids. I am unrepentant about my refusal to go. In the department we did not neglect the other health issues, but at that point Aids needed very direct political intervention. I was immensely helped here by the two men to whom I dedicate this book. The effort also established one other point. Over the 1980s we had had one health policy dispute after another. Aids showed just what the health service could achieve when we were all working on the same side. I am afraid none of these arguments convinced the Iron Lady, and Aids remained conspicuously absent from the memoirs of her years at No. 10.

I should make one point clear. I do not claim that Britain was unique in the early action we took to combat the Aids pandemic. There were other countries making similar efforts. If you had travelled to Sydney at that time you would have found a vigorous public education campaign beginning and, in the years that followed, you would have seen determined efforts to stem the spread of the disease. In India there would be a prevention campaign which culminated in the formation of a special organisation to combat Aids; and in Berlin and Amsterdam there were enormous efforts to communicate with drug users and not isolate them. The United States might have been doing little in public education but financially they were devoting more money to research than any other country. In Europe, France also was putting emphasis on research. So I neither claim international leadership nor that Britain was successful in every aspect of policy. Take testing in prisons. Back in 1986 I commented approvingly in my diary that the Home Secretary refused to be stampeded into instant decisions on this. I should have known better. The idea of stampeding the Home Office into anything is highly optimistic. In the end, it took them almost thirty years to stumble to a policy on testing.

What I do claim is rather different. By an early stage in the epidemic, without the help of drugs or a vaccine, we knew what could work. We knew that publicity could bring home to people the dangers. We knew it could alter attitudes and successfully promote the use of condoms. Those results were also established at the centre of the worldwide epidemic in sub-Saharan Africa when Uganda (ironically, given their later performance) ran effective public health publicity, notably with their ABC campaign – Abstain, Be faithful, use a Condom. It also became clear in country after country that the struggle to introduce clean needles and substitute methadone was achieving dramatic success. The figures from around the world could not have been clearer. Even at that early stage there was evidence that could have been used to stem the disease.

But of course Margaret Thatcher was not alone among political leaders of the 1980s and 1990s in looking the other way. As a political issue Aids promised few rewards. There was the potential embarrassment of becoming involved in intricate issues of sexual health, while the good being done was to groups who were not notably popular – gays, lesbians, drug users and sex workers. Surely, too many leaders thought, a few local campaigns could settle the matter? Millions of deaths later, the answer to that question is obvious, but at the time Ronald Reagan in the United States refused to acknowledge the seriousness of the position and turned the other way. Even worse, in South Africa Nelson Mandela may have guided his nation through its first post-apartheid government, but he failed to respond to the tragedy that was enveloping his country. Margaret Thatcher may have grumbled but, with the exception of the cancelled ministerial broadcast, she did not veto our efforts. Albeit reluctantly, she allowed me to get on with the job.

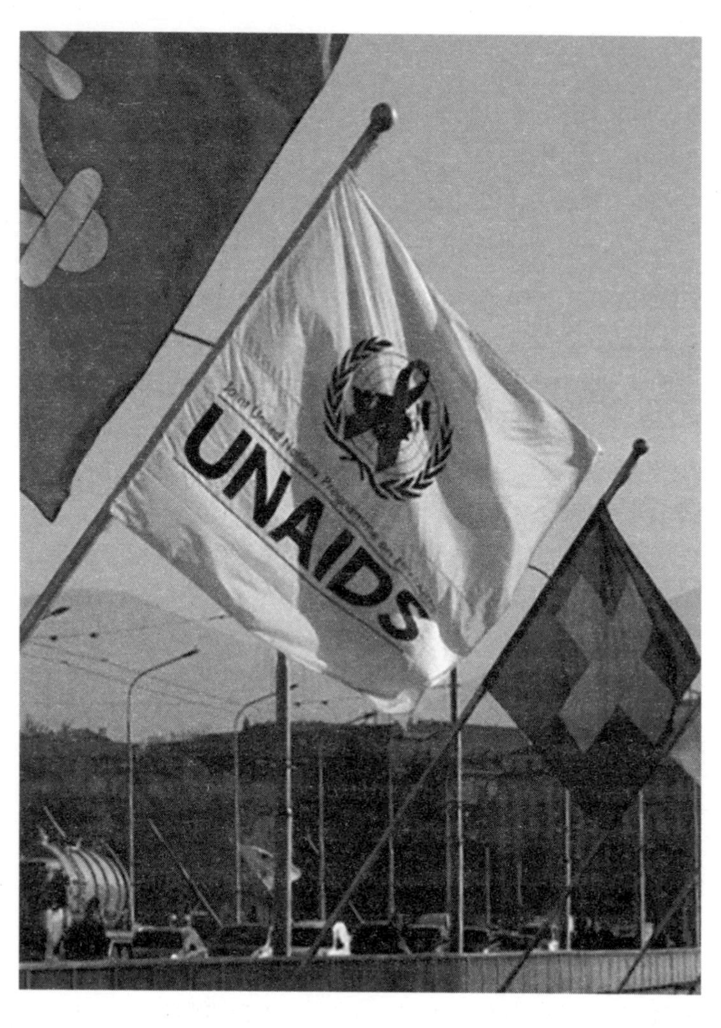

A UNAIDS flag flies in the health capital of the world.

TWO

GENEVA: THE TIPPING POINT

SWITZERLAND MAY SEEM a curious country to start my travels. What can this eminently respectable and sedate nation know of HIV and Aids and the human problems they cause? The answer is that they know rather more than you might think. For example, during the brief period between 1987 and 1992 Zurich, and more particularly the Platzspitz Park next to the Swiss National Museum, offered clean needles and syringes to all comers and a freedom from prosecution while in the park. The idea was to tackle the burgeoning drug problem in the city and with it the spread of HIV and Aids. You could call it an experiment ahead of its time. In fact, it was a badly organised scheme which acted as a magnet for both drug users and pushers alike. Drug users (many from outside Switzerland) flocked to take advantage of what became known as 'needle park' and in 1992 the scheme was finally closed down. But I did not visit Switzerland to look in detail at the history of Zurich's needle park or the challenge it faces today – except to register in passing that every country in the world faces a drugs problem and solutions need more than good intentions. Rather my intention is to travel two hours, thirty-eight minutes by Switzerland's impeccably punctual trains to Geneva, which stands near the border with France. For, if any city can lay claim to be the health capital of the world, it is Geneva.

Clustered on a campus a few miles from the city centre with distant views of a range of snow-capped mountains is the massive headquarters of the World Health Organization. Formed after the Second World War in 1948, but with roots in the pre-war League of Nations, it is the specialist health agency of the United Nations. Facing it in a tower of long corridors is UNAIDS, which was started in 1996 specifically to give a new impetus to the battle against HIV and Aids. Back across the tree-lined oblong of lawn which divides the campus is the newest health body on the block: UNITAID, formed in 2006 with the aim of ensuring affordable medicines and getting the best value for money out of the billions of dollars now spent on tackling HIV and a range of other health conditions. They are temporarily, but appropriately, housed in portable cabins. A short distance away down the road towards the lake is the headquarters of the International

Red Cross, while away from the campus altogether is an anonymous office building that houses the Global Fund to Fight Aids, Tuberculosis and Malaria, which gathers in money from governments around the world and distributes about $4 billion a year in aid directed at HIV (where 60 per cent of their budget goes) as well as at malaria and tuberculosis. There is no better place than Geneva to get a view of the history and advance of HIV and Aids around the world and the value of the measures taken to check it.

From a fairly early stage we knew how HIV was passed. As one of our British health leaflets said in the autumn of 1986, 'all proven cases have been caused by semen or blood'. Shared needles was the blood route; sexual intercourse (gay or straight) was the seminal route and the one that caused most casualties. There never was any logical reason to believe, as many claimed back then, that HIV was somehow *exclusively* a 'gay disease'. Although in the 1980s the wards in San Francisco were full of dying gay men, the hospitals in parts of West Africa were packed with young women. Given the widespread homophobia in most African countries, any suggestion that gay sex was a large scale means of transmission was fiercely denied.

Peter Piot, who later was to become the first director general of UNAIDS, tells a story in his autobiography *No Time to Lose* of meeting a general from Zaire (now the Democratic Republic of the Congo) whose clothes were literally hanging off his body and who obviously had

Aids. He was proud of his sexual prowess and boasted of the many, many notches on his belt. 'Naturally I'm a real man,' he said. 'A real man needs women, many women.' Tentatively Piot suggested that he might also from time to time have had sex with a man. 'What!' Bellowed the general. 'Never. How can you even think that. How filthy. How deranged.'

Piot worked in West Africa as an epidemiologist in the 1970s and made his name with his contribution to identifying the Ebola virus, which was uncovered in 1976 following reports that several Belgian nuns working in a hospital in Zaire had died from a mystery infection. Many more died before it was tracked down to the hospital itself and the lethally poor hygiene there. In an uncanny forerunner of HIV, the researchers found that the sharing of infected syringes had spread the epidemic.

A few years after the first Ebola cases, the first cases of Aids were *officially* recognised. In 1981 there was an American report that five young gay white men in Los Angeles had contracted a mystery illness and later that year the medical correspondent of *The Times* in London reported that 'an unexplained epidemic of infections and cancer among young male homosexuals is causing growing concern in medical circles'. Only one death had been reported in London but in the United States the figures had shot up during the year with 180 reported cases and seventy deaths. The report added that homosexuals who had developed the disease had been found 'to give very low responses to standard tests of their immune systems – a condition known medically as being immuno-compromised. That has led American doctors to name the condition the 'gay compromise syndrome'.

It was the beginning of the flood, but were these actually the first cases? Few believe that. There may be disagreement about just when the first cases occurred, but there is general agreement that it was long before the headlines of the 1980s. One apparently certain earlier case was unearthed by Michael Worobey, an American ecologist, while he was working in West Africa. He reasoned that unexplained deaths exhibiting symptoms which were later identified as Aids almost certainly would have led doctors in the 1950s and 1960s to have ordered biopsies. It was just possible that some of these biopsies might have survived – and so it proved. At the university of Kinshasa, wax encased biopsy samples had been stored carefully away. Finally, after months of painstaking research, he discovered remnants of HIV in a tissue taken from a 28-year-old woman who had died in 1960. Some researchers believe that there are earlier cases also waiting to be verified.

But where did it come from? To my mind the most convincing theory on the origin of HIV is put forward by Timberg and Halperin in their 2012 book *Tinderbox*. Roughly condensed, it is that the HIV had been slowly spreading unnoticed, perhaps for decades, before the first cases came to official notice. Genetically, HIV closely resembles strains of the virus SIV (simian immunodeficiency virus) found in chimpanzees, and therefore it was reasonable to think that there could be a link. In West Africa, chimpanzees are sold by the side of the road as bush meat and what could have happened is that a man became infected, through an open wound, either when picking up the bloody animal he had just hunted or in preparing the animal for sale. Either way, the man became infected with the virus and in turn he sexually infected others. The long, long route of global transmission began.

At first, Timberg and Halperin suggest, the virus was contained locally in a remote part of Cameroon but gradually, in the colonial years of Africa and afterwards, the virus spread more widely. Some of those who had been infected locally travelled down the Congo River to what was then Leopoldville and is now Kinshasa. The big city facilitated the spread and from there the virus went by road to neighbouring parts of Africa. But how did it travel to the United States? The simplest explanation is by ship and by infected seamen to the West Coast of the United States, perhaps to a port city like San Francisco. Another branch of basically the same theory gives Haiti an unwilling part in the story. After the Belgians withdrew abruptly and without preparation from the Congo in 1960, there was a need for professional groups, like teachers and engineers, that the colonial power had failed so lamentably to train locally. Some of these posts were eagerly filled by well-educated Haitians anxious to escape for a while the notorious rule of François ('Papa Doc') Duvalier. When they returned to Haiti (on holiday or more permanently) that country became a HIV staging post to the New World.

Outside the world of epidemiology all this sounds fairly extraordinary if not fanciful. Who has ever heard of the biggest epidemic to strike the world in modern times being caused by some harmless chimps in an under-populated part of Cameroon? Is it really possible that they could have been the root of an infection which wiped out men and women by the million throughout sub-Saharan Africa as well as gay men in the bath houses of San Francisco and the drug users in the slums of Moscow? Surely it defies belief? But then you have to remember the history of other viruses. In the 1960s the Marburg virus was identified after a number of pharmaceutical workers in Germany had been infected by a batch of monkeys imported from Uganda. Seven of the twenty-five who had been in direct contact with the monkeys died. One trace takes the Marburg infection back to cave-dwelling African fruit bats and suspicion also falls on them as the root cause of the Ebola virus. As for the wider communication to the general population, we should remember that the Great Plague of the seventeenth century was spread by fleas on the backs of rats. In modern times there is no better way of sending a virus around the globe than through sex and drugs.

Whatever the explanation, there is no doubt about the sheer speed of the next stage. Between 1981 and 2000 the number of people living with HIV around the world increased from less than one million to over twenty-seven million. Sub-Saharan Africa was the very worst affected, with around a quarter of the population infected in some countries, but most other countries have also felt the impact. Deaths rose to alarming and tragic heights and antiretroviral drugs were still in short supply. At the same time the theories of the denialists that HIV was not the cause of Aids, or that it was an epidemic that affected only gay men, were shot full of holes. In Britain in the 1980s I was often accused of overreacting to the danger. Given that it was a virus which spread so rapidly, which could kill so many and had no cure, and what has happened around the world since then, I am amazed at my moderation.

Aids could have been checked early, but the world was tragically slow to recognise what was happening and even slower to do anything substantial about it. As one WHO official told me, 'We allowed the tragedy to explode before our eyes.' In the 1980s and 1990s the developing public health crisis was clear for anyone who wanted to see but many of the countries it most severely affected were largely out of sight of the rich West. In particular they were the African countries south of the Sahara desert that did not have the resources or the health systems to tackle such an epidemic. In truth they desperately needed international help – although perversely some African nations refused to recognise the monster that was at their door and even rejected help when it was offered. The result was that the most basic and cheapest prevention tool – the male condom – remained largely unavailable in the countries where the epidemic was expanding the fastest. The efficacy of circumcision as a substantial, but not total, protection had yet to be recognised. The plight of injecting drug users and sex workers was widely ignored – as it still is. The resources devoted to the fight were hopelessly inadequate.

Sir Richard Feachem, the founding director of the Global Fund, said that in the 1990s,

> *the global epidemic raged unabated. It was almost as if humankind had decided to conduct a large natural experiment. 'Let's see what happens if we all deliberately decide to do nothing and let the virus take its natural course.' What happened was devastating. Massive national, regional and global epidemics, cutting decades from life expectancy in southern Africa and crippling economies and welfare in many countries.*

A similar perspective comes from Peter Piot. Looking back to 1995, when he started UNAIDS, he says:

> *It was clear to me that the response to Aids was woefully inadequate. Low and middle income countries*

were spending just $250 million a year and only two, Uganda and Thailand, had achieved even modest reductions in new infections. There was no coordination between United Nations agencies, no involvement of civil organisations outside high income countries, people living with HIV battled stigma and discrimination, and there was no effective treatment.

UNAIDS started to improve the position slowly. The first priority was to get better estimates of the scale of the disaster. Up to then the collection system was fairly rudimentary. One country insisted in putting in its return in pencil and, more seriously, countries like Russia, South Africa and India accused the agency of exaggerating the epidemic. As it happened, in 2007 UNAIDS was forced to concede that in a number of countries, including India, they had indeed overstated the figures. I remember being in New Delhi at the time that the Indian figures were downgraded – to an almost audible sigh of official satisfaction. Today UNAIDS says that it now asks for and receives much more detailed information. Dr Peter Ghys, the director of epidemic monitoring, says that the figures rest on 'much more data both in quantity and quality'.

What these figures show is that the first decade of the twenty-first century was a period of undoubted progress. Antiretroviral drugs had first appeared in 1986 as single agents with limited efficacy. By 1996 highly active antiretroviral therapy using multiple drugs in combination became available but at sky-high prices. Slowly, as prices came down, they became more available to people in the developing world. At the same time they became dramatically easier to take. Rather than a cocktail of perhaps twenty pills taken at the same time, by 2010 patients needed to take only one – although this pill still contained three different compounds. UNAIDS played a valuable role in this development but the real game-changers were the start of the Global Fund in 2002 and the President's Fund in the United States (PEPFAR) the year following. From this point big resources began to flow.

Ironically the Global Fund to Fight Aids, Tuberculosis and Malaria was a product of the 2001 meeting of the G8 assembly of the top economic nations in Genoa, where 200,000 anti-globalisation protesters battled with brutal Italian riot police. Richard Feachem (in words which would have been approved by most of the Genoa demonstrators) said of the meeting 'We were driven by the passion and anger of the advocates, activists and affected communities. Business as usual was clearly not going to do the job. Something new, different and far more impactful was required.'

The Global Fund was a new step in that it put responsibility on the nation asking for help to put forward the schemes they thought most important, rather than having it decided for them. 'No longer would young and inexperienced staff members of agencies in Washington,

London or Geneva dream up what was best for Malawi,' Feachem says. 'Ownership of programmes, of success and of failure, would lie with the country and not with the Global Fund.' In its first five years the fund raised around $11 billion and supported projects in 140 countries.

So where does the world stand today? Not surprisingly, in Geneva health officials argue that they have made massive progress – and they have. The rapid expansion of antiretroviral therapy (ART) is rightly claimed as one of the most remarkable achievements in public health history. The drugs now reach over ten million people around the world, which is a twentyfold increase since 2003. In Africa in 2000 very few received treatment (0.1 per cent); today treatment is provided for over 40 per cent who are judged to need it.[1] Deaths are almost a quarter lower than their 2005 peak and life expectancy has risen significantly in a whole range of countries. New infections have reduced by a fifth since the turn of the century and there are many fewer babies born with HIV.

In a few short years the President's Fund from the United States and the Global Fund from Geneva have grown to become by far the biggest donors of aid for HIV in the world. Although they are frequently not given credit for it, the American contribution dwarfs all else. It not only gives directly through PEPFAR and USAID, it

1. This is on the pre-2013 WHO definition of when treatment should begin, which I will discuss later in this chapter.

provides almost a third of the Global Fund's resources; America is precluded from giving more on the basis, so it is said, that if they did the rest of the world might sit back and leave them to it. As it is, Britain and France are the Fund's next biggest contributors (Britain having doubled its contribution in 2013) but rich countries like Germany and Japan inexplicably lag far behind. A range of other international organisations such as the World Bank also make contributions together with a never-to-be-forgotten small army of civil society organisations such as those of Bill and Melinda Gates, George Soros, Elton John and Bill Clinton, together with Médecins Sans Frontières, the International HIV Alliance, the International Aids Vaccine Initiative and many, many more. Global HIV investment from all sources in 2012 was almost $19 billion – a tenfold increase since 2001. An even more hopeful trend is the way that national governments that have in the past been recipients of outside aid are increasingly taking responsibility for their own populations. South Africa now claims to finance 80 per cent of its treatment spending.

To sum up this progress, I will quote one senior WHO doctor who suddenly revealed his credo. 'We have an extraordinary opportunity,' he said.

> *We have established what can be done. We have delivered programmes in refugee camps and in townships. We have shown you can eliminate mother to child transmission. There has never been a time when*

> *we have seen the development of so many new medicines in so short a time or seen so many organisations working together. When you compare HIV with other public health conditions like tuberculosis you know how far we have come.*

He is right. The *opportunity* is there. The progress that has been made is dramatic. The lives that have been saved represent a magnificent achievement. Equally, we should be in no doubt about the debit side of the balance sheet. Deaths may be down from their peak of 2.5 million a year but the toll is still an appalling 1.6 million a year. New HIV infections continue to outpace new treatment. The South Africans may be increasingly providing for themselves, but many other countries have not followed suit. Many nations rely almost entirely on outside support when financing schemes for drug users, sex workers or men having sex with men. Ministers don't like getting involved in such potentially embarrassing and unpopular areas.

Yet it is precisely in these 'key populations' where we need to make progress. A UNAIDS survey in 2012 showed that, in forty-nine countries that produced data, the prevalence of HIV among injecting drug users was at least twenty times greater than in the general population, and in eleven of them prevalence was at least fifty-fold higher. Yet prejudice against drug users and the mistaken belief that harm-reduction policies increase crime means that clean needles and methadone can become a government 'no go' area. Even when countries have such programmes, the supply of clean needles can be sparse. In the measured words of UNAIDS, 'The world is far from being on track to achieve the global target.' Or – to put it more bluntly – despite all the advances, we are failing.

Some would argue that there is some underlying sympathy with drug users. Most middle-class families in the West (and not just the West) have had some experience of it through children, relations or friends. Not many have escaped. Men having sex with men, on the other hand, often raises an almost primeval response. In many parts of the globe homosexual men are ostracised, discriminated against, and assaulted. They become easy prey for blackmail and extortion. When he wrote about equal marriage in 2013 Dr Carey, the former Archbishop of Canterbury, talked of Christians in Britain becoming 'a persecuted minority'. If the noble prelate wants to see a real persecuted minority he should look to the gay community.

To a greater or lesser extent discrimination is the experience of millions of gay men, lesbians and transgender people around the world. They are not loved and too many governments follow the public. Ministers know that such minorities are not a popular cause in their countries and they can safely look the other way. At best their attitude is that if international bodies want to provide testing and treatment, then that is up to them and it saves governments the embarrassment of even trying to persuade their own public to support such policies. And that is precisely what happens. The figures from Geneva show that in low- and middle-income countries no less than 92 per cent of the finance to tackle this obvious issue of public health is provided from international sources. The receiving countries could hardly show their distaste for the groups most vulnerable to HIV more clearly.

In almost eighty countries homosexuality is a crime which leaves gay people open to prosecution and imprisonment – even the threat of execution. It will be a brave man who comes forward for testing in one of those countries and risks exposure to the law. The public health result is bad for him and bad for others – most often wives and partners – as the virus is spread further. Some apologists claim that often the law is not enforced rigorously – as if this prevents corrupt police and officials from extracting money, or does away with the stigma that surrounds gay sex, or indeed does anything for public health.

And then there is sex work. Even its name raises controversy. In London one minister insisted that all references in a sexual health paper which had referred to 'sex workers' should be changed to 'prostitutes'. In Geneva they prefer 'sex work' and if you want cooperation from sex workers then it is a more sensible description – and you do need cooperation if for no other reason than the fact that, in the precise words of UNAIDS, 'female sex workers are 13.5 times more likely to be living with HIV than are other women'. That of course is an average across the world; it misses out the sky high rates in countries like Swaziland (70 per cent), Guinea Bissau (40 per cent) and Uganda (36 per cent).

The law round the world is equivocal. Sex work is illegal but tolerated. Almost everywhere there are legal restrictions but almost everywhere the police turn a blind eye or, just as likely, take protection payment from the sex workers. Corruption bedevils the whole area but no one much cares. On national agendas sex workers come low, if not last, in the table of priorities. In Kiev, for example, the leader of the sex workers' association had never met a government minister and was embarrassingly overjoyed to be photographed with an ex-minister like me.

There are other issues also that need to be tackled but may well offend the more sensitive. An obvious example is sex in prisons. The first bridge to get over is that it happens at all – which it self-evidently does. So what are the consequences for policy? One is the provision of condoms which is now accepted in most sensible countries although, for some reason, testing for HIV (even on a voluntary basis) is often still regarded as a step too far. This is in spite of the evidence from Washington DC that the vast majority of prisoners raise no objection.

As for antiretroviral treatment the impact has been obviously hugely beneficial but we should never forget the excluded. For the last decade the guidance from the

WHO was that antiretroviral treatment should be started when the CD4 lymphocyte count in the blood went below 350 cells per micro litre of blood. The CD4 count of the average reasonably healthy HIV-free person is between 600 and 1,000. The major danger of serious life-threatening complications from HIV comes when the CD4 count falls below 200. The WHO has now reviewed this limit and the 2013 guideline is that those with HIV should start treatment not at 350 but when the CD4 count falls below 500. That changes the goal posts substantially and means that, in spite of all the progress, only a third of the twenty-eight million people with HIV living in low- and middle-income countries are now receiving antiretroviral treatment when they need it.

Children are particularly disadvantaged. Extraordinarily, they receive proportionately less antiretroviral treatment than adults and that position is unlikely to change soon. Of approaching seventeen million children who have lost one or both parents to Aids, almost fifteen million are African. A further unwelcome trend is that in several countries there is now an increase in risky behaviour – men and women taking more partners, a decline in the use of condoms, even the sharing of needles under the influence of so-called recreational drugs. The assumption, particularly of users in the prosperous West, is that antiretroviral drugs are available and so even if they do contract HIV they can still look forward to a long and unrestricted life. The risk of HIV does not hold the same terror as before. Perhaps the prevention message is all too often failing or – even more likely – has never been seriously attempted.

It is difficult to avoid the conclusion that, in spite of all the brave words about the bright future, the world still remains in crisis, and a quick tour of the statistics and policies on prevention, information and treatment around the world at present bears this out. Africa is still at the epicentre of the epidemic. As UNAIDS says, 'There is always one piece of the pie chart that is biggest, one vertical column that is tallest, one trend line that is steepest: Africa.' Out of the thirty-six million people who are living with HIV no fewer than twenty-five million live in Africa, predominantly south of the Sahara. In South Africa six million live with HIV, in Nigeria the figure is almost 3.4 million and in Kenya over 1.5 million. Overall in the countries of sub-Saharan Africa almost one in twenty adults live with HIV. In some African countries prevalence among sex workers is nearly 40 per cent and new infections among men having sex with men run at almost 20 per cent. The promotion of basic prevention measures like the condom range from patchy to non-existent. Even President Museveni's much praised ABC campaign in Uganda – 'Abstain, be Faithful, use a Condom'– is a pale shadow of what it used to be.

In Asia, India has over two million people living with HIV (although this is out of a population of over a billion) while in Indonesia the figure is over 600,000 and in Thailand 440,000. But we should not ignore some of the encouraging signs. Cambodia, for example, claims to have achieved universal access to antiretroviral treatment, while Thailand's figures are a substantial improvement on ten years ago. Thailand's work in providing condoms for sex workers rightly comes in for praise – as does the exuberance of some of the campaigning – but there is another side to the Thai coin. Like another ten countries in the region it threatens the death penalty for drug offences. UNAIDS summarises the gains across the Asian region as 'insufficient and fragile'.

Elsewhere, stony-faced policies on drug users mean that in Eastern and Central Europe the rate of HIV infection continues to grow. UNAIDS estimates that half the new infections are because of drug users sharing needles. If any further proof was needed of the failure of the old Soviet policies in handling intravenous drug use you only need to look at the comparison between East and West. In Eastern European countries like Belarus, Georgia and Moldova the position continues to deteriorate, while in Western Europe (where clean-needle policies are now commonplace) infection has stabilised at a very low level. Western Europe generally has lower HIV prevalence but there is still a heavy price to be paid in those countries. Britain for example has 100,000 people living with HIV, which in drugs and care alone costs the health service about £1 billion a year and rising.

In the largely Muslim countries of the Middle East and North Africa there have been significant, and potentially ominous, increases. Although the numbers are comparatively small, it gives the lie to the assertion that men having sex with men 'never happens here'. In Latin America it is estimated that about 1.4 million people live with HIV, with the biggest numbers in the drug affected countries of Mexico (170,000) and Colombia (150,000). The region with the highest infection rate after Africa is the Caribbean, with 1 per cent prevalence and Haiti accounting for over half the cases.

And then there is China. The official figures show around 800,000 people living with HIV, although some would put the number at over a million. In 2009 China reported that Aids had become the leading cause of death from infectious diseases for the first time, and later reports have shown that heterosexual sex is the dominant form of transmission. The result has been that over the last ten years China has made much more serious efforts to contain the virus than in the years before, which were characterised by denial and inaction. Clean needles and methadone have been introduced and 2007 saw the first major television campaign to promote condom use – twenty years late but notably successful. Even so, attitudes generally have taken longer to change. There was an attempt in 2013 to ban those with HIV from public baths and there continue to be stories of medical treatment being refused. Sex work exists in a kind of no man's land. One health worker described it to me. On his way to work in the morning he would pass a number of brothels.

The women would wave to passers-by from the windows but when there was a major ceremonial visit the brothels were closed – only to open again as soon as the visiting dignitary had left.

At this point I should perhaps make something clear. My purpose is not to attempt a comprehensive and detailed description of the position in every country of the world. UNAIDS does this admirably in its annual reports. My aim in visiting some of the major cities around the globe is to draw out some of the common issues that affect us all, to propose the policies we need if we are to make progress and to describe the main obstacles that stand in the way of bringing the epidemic under control. Of course I have not been everywhere and I make no apology for that. To attempt such a task would not only be gigantic but would put you out of date at one end of the world by the time you have reached the other. Even as it was, the political position in Ukraine changed out of all recognition from my first visit to the next, and is changing still.

In Geneva there is no doubt about how they see the way forward: give us the money and we will finish the job. In the words of one international worker there, 'If the resources are available we can do wonders.' The trouble is that it is a big '*if*'. There can hardly have been a worse time to ask for more resources than the last seven or eight years. International aid is not a popular cause at any time, let alone at a time of recession. Almost inevitably the cry goes up 'what about us?' Often it comes from people whose standard of living is infinitely higher than that of the grindingly poor, who are the usual beneficiaries of help overseas. Nevertheless, many politicians and newspapers see it as an all too obvious target for cuts. Their campaigns are aided by charges of official corruption and funds misapplied. And it can hardly be denied that even a cursory reading of the local press as you travel the world shows just how widespread that corruption appears to be, and that it certainly stretches into taking money intended for the sick and the dying.

We have seen one round of fund-raising abandoned by the Global Fund for lack of international support, while at the same time international resources for low- and middle-income countries have stopped increasing in real terms. This is of immense importance. As the Kaiser Family Foundation, which has been reviewing international assistance for HIV since 2002, comment in their 2013 report, 'In the last decade donor governments drove a dramatic increase in funding scale-up, which helped to turn the tide of the epidemic. Yet donor funding has plateaued since the global economic turndown in 2008 and does not show signs of increasing.' In other words, help has been frozen. Perhaps now, with the partial international recovery, conditions for giving will improve. Perhaps.

The trouble is that, historically, donor countries have seen giving money for HIV and Aids as different from helping other health conditions in one important respect. For most conditions, a single course of treatment will normally be sufficient. Even if it takes six or twelve months, the cured patient will make way for a new patient inside the budget. With HIV the position is radically different. HIV is a lifetime condition requiring a lifetime of treatment and, with present knowledge, a lifetime's supply of drugs. As one Geneva official honestly conceded, 'On present knowledge you need to keep people on treatment for the next forty years.' Or, as I used to repeat time and time again back in the 1980s, 'There is no vaccine; there is no cure.'

From the financial point of view this has clear consequences. Once you have placed people with HIV on treatment you cannot take them off and the likelihood is that they will need more care, not less, as their lives progress. The drugs bill could well increase. UNAIDS say, 'As drug resistance increases over time more patients will require second and third generation medicines. Most of these more recent medicines will remain under patent for years to come resulting in potentially drastic increases in treatment costs.'

So what happens if you continue to freeze spending at its present historically high figure? It may sound eminently reasonable to hard-pressed finance ministers, but what it means in reality is that the epidemic will be given new legs. If you leave people untreated then the virus will have the opportunity to continue to spread. This is what happens in epidemics. This is how we got into this mess in the first place. It will mean more deaths, more suffering, more orphans and all the other human consequences that go with a failure of policy. Rather than meeting the UNAIDS target of reducing the utterly unacceptable total of 2.3 million new infections a year to 500,000, the danger is that the process could even go into reverse. The world would have given up much of the ground so painfully won over the last decade.

What we should do is to see how we can increase the treatment for those living with HIV while at the same time preventing the further spread of the virus. We need to know at what point the use of antiretroviral drugs benefits the public generally. One proposal is to go beyond even the WHO's new guidance and in effect say that antiretroviral drugs should be given as early as possible as a prevention intervention. The point is this: if you leave the person with HIV untreated then he or she is infectious to others and the virus spreads. If the person with HIV starts effective antiretroviral therapy at the time of diagnosis and this is successfully sustained for the long term, then there is a real prospect that onward transmission could fall dramatically. That is the case made by those who advocate antiretroviral treatment as a means of prevention. They say that if antiretroviral treatment can be given as quickly as possible after a patient is found to be HIV positive that in itself will reduce the spread. Their claim is that prevention can cut onward transmission dramatically – by over 90 per cent. The point is given added emphasis in that HIV is dramatically at its most infectious immediately after acquisition.

But surely the cost of introducing such an ambitious policy would be prohibitive? The reply to that is that, in the end, everyone who has HIV will need antiretroviral drugs. What you are doing is bringing the cost forward, but with the bonus that if the policy is successful then new cases will reduce and the numbers of new infections will fall. Finance ministers will not like the cost being pushed forward, but the prospective gain for national exchequers and for public health in reducing the pool of those with HIV is obvious. There is also another bonus. As some of the antiretrovirals come off patent there will be the opportunity for cheaper generics. The newer medicines will remain on patent but some of the older (but proven) drugs will not. There is a once in a generation opportunity to achieve substantially lower drug prices.

But if we are to pursue such a radically new policy there are two conditions. First, those without HIV need to continue (or start) to take sensible precautions. All the old messages about using a condom, sticking to one partner and not sharing needles apply today. There is a shared responsibility in preventing HIV and governments must try anew to get this message across. Second, we need as a matter of urgency to reduce the vast number of people with HIV who are undiagnosed. Even in rich countries like the United States and Britain the number of undiagnosed is over a fifth of the total and in many other countries the proportion is much, much higher. As it stands, no policy, old or new, will reach them. The undiagnosed are not only a danger to themselves but a massive public health danger to everybody else. The need throughout the world is for more effective testing policies which also spell out the advantages of treatment.

The real decision for governments is whether we are prepared to switch to a policy of treatment *and* prevention, or bump along with the present policy of treating casualties while allowing fresh men and women to be infected. The question is where you put the interests of public health generally. Will we ever win the battle against HIV if we do not give prevention an infinitely higher priority? As it happens, a policy of ensuring that antiretrovirals are available for everyone who has HIV, irrespective of their CD4 count, holds out promise for both the patients and the public generally.

If I was to attempt an interim judgement, I would say that the world has come a long way but it now stands on the edge. We know the problems and we have shown that we can master most of them. The question is: have we the will to see it through? Have we the will to tackle the stigma and prejudice which gets in the way of so much progress? Have we the will to increase the financial support? Those questions need urgent reply. Over the next pages I will report on the response from eight further cities of the world: from Entebbe and Cape Town in sub--Saharan Africa at the epicentre of the epidemic; from the old Cold War capitals of Washington and Moscow together with Kiev, once a Russian satellite; from New Delhi, with its massive population and Sydney with its surprisingly pragmatic policies; and then back to Europe and London, where I first began. We might remember that in the world generally population trends are not in our favour. We can expect an increase in the world population of one and a half billion over the next twenty years. There will be more sexually active young people year by year. The dismal lack of sex education around the world will mean that many will be unprepared and ignorant.

To my mind the job is at best only half done. We still have countries that are in effect in denial, vulnerable groups that are surrounded at every turn by stigma and prejudice, governments that have lost some of the determination to succeed and have relapsed into complacency and a resistance to doing self-evident good. Too often the debate has changed. Rather than 'What can we do to help?' the question has become 'Is this aid really necessary?' In the West, Aids has too often slipped off the public and political agenda and 'is it still a problem?' is a startlingly common question. In writing this book I have been struck by just how many people in the West think that it is yesterday's issue. We need to wake up to what is happening around the world. Unless we do we face continued human disaster. New efforts, new resources and new policies are urgently needed if we are not to go backwards. Today we are at a tipping point.

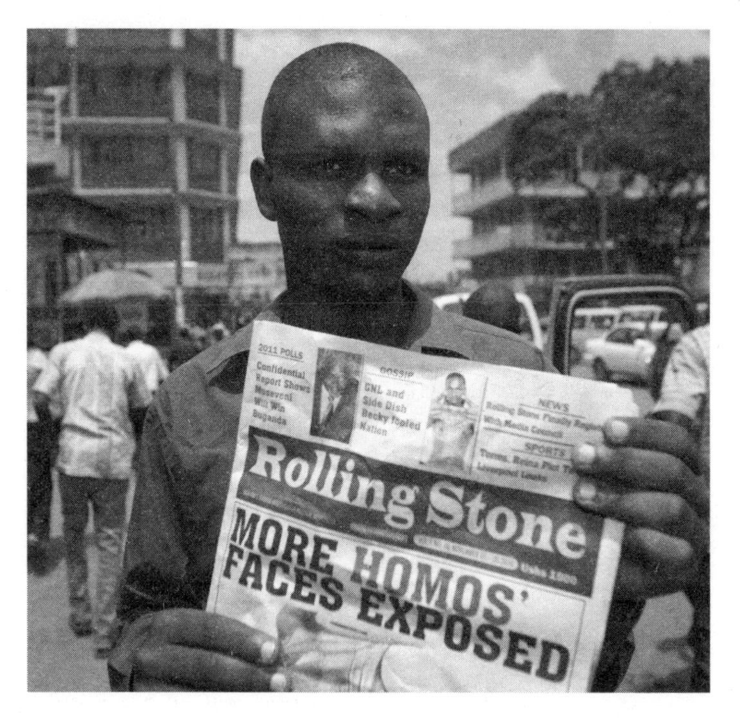

The notorious Rolling Stone *newspaper, which specialised in 'exposing' gay men, putting them in danger of attack.*

THREE

ENTEBBE: THE GOOD, THE BAD AND THE UGLY

ENTEBBE HAS SEVERAL faces. The best remembered dates back to 1976 when the airport was the scene of one of the most daring hostage release operations of the twentieth century. Israeli commandos stormed the airport's terminal building, freeing over 100 hostages but in the process killing over twenty Ugandan troops who, on the orders of President Idi Amin, were backing the kidnappers rather than the kidnapped. On the Israeli side there was one casualty – the leader of the raid, Colonel Yonatan Netanyahu – the elder brother of Israel's future Prime Minister. Today, the traveller to Entebbe is welcomed (yes, welcomed) by smiling immigration staff. When he moves to one of the hotels that line the shores of Lake Victoria (the second largest lake in the world and about the size of Ireland) he looks out on an immense, apparently gentle blue expanse of softly undulating water. Palm trees grow in well-tended green gardens and Marabou storks glide gracefully in the sky above. All seems well with the world.

At Entebbe hospital a few miles down the road the picture is rather different. The hospital is a straggle of low buildings with red corrugated iron roofs. As the temperature begins to rise in the wards, patients stretch out or sit listlessly on beds which have been moved close together. It is the only way of ensuring that a hospital built at the time of the First World War can, a century later, meet the vastly increased demand. The maternity unit alone delivers 400 to 500 babies a month in a country where the majority of the population is under eighteen. But it is HIV which causes the greatest pressure on the overworked and brave staff.

The coolest place in the hospital is the room where blood samples are stored, but even so achieving testing results is not easy. Testing kits can run out as the financial year progresses and many who should be tested either ignore the calls to come in or simply find the journey too difficult or too expensive. Others who do test leave it dangerously late. They may be wives who have kept their HIV secret from their husbands in fear of the violence and ostracism that awaits them. Or they may be business people who fear the consequences if their condition becomes known. When I visited there in January 2013, one of the hospital staff told me: 'The more educated they are, the less willing they are to come forward.' In one case a doctor presented himself when his illness was so advanced that he might just as well have gone straight to the undertaker.

In Entebbe hospital money is short. The hospital has not received a budget increase from the health ministry for over a decade – partly as a result of the endemic corruption which has seen too much outside aid intended for health care siphoned off. Nevertheless the hospital dispenses antiretroviral drugs for free – although it is estimated that nationwide only about half of those who need drug treatment receive it, which explains why the death toll from Aids is still around 65,000 a year. The further prevention measure of male circumcision is now making some progress in spite of critics who say that it simply encourages promiscuity. A poster outside the small operating room shows a wife saying, 'I am proud I have a circumcised husband because we have less chance of getting HIV.' Advocates of circumcision like Timberg and Halperin say that their case is established in a range of African countries. The reason is simple enough. The skin on the shaft of a man's penis is relatively thick and tough allowing it to serve as a natural barrier against infection but the foreskin of an uncircumcised man is unusually vulnerable because it is soft, thin and a bit moist, making it easier for pathogens to penetrate. The only difficulty is persuading those who have been circumcised that it is not a guarantee against contracting HIV – just a help. But help of any kind is desperately needed in Uganda.

About an hour's drive from Entebbe, the last miles down a rutted unmade road, is one of the fishing villages of Lake Victoria. Here fishermen land their catches and the people from the islands which dot Lake Victoria come in to buy their stores. It might sound like another tourist destination but it is anything but that. It is a shanty town where life is brutal and only the fittest survive. The shacks are cheek by jowl with each other and narrow unmade paths lead through the jumble. From inside one of the hovels there is the noise of men drinking. Outside, a naked baby sits unattended in the dirt. It is all reminiscent of an eighteenth-century Hogarth cartoon. On the shore men wade into the water to carry in the islanders who have made their way over in long, roughly built canoe-like boats with outboards. The porters spend their days in the water to scratch a living with goodness knows what consequences to their own health. In the background a giant rubbish dump smoulders slowly. As for the fishermen themselves, life is difficult and can be dangerous. They fish at night, the lake can become dangerously rough, safety measures are virtually non-existent and many of the fishermen cannot swim. Their earnings are low but the sale of the fish gives them cash in hand. They spend their days drinking, gambling and, of course, having sex.

To meet the demand this small, sad outpost of humanity has its own distinct red-light district with incongruous lines of washing drying in the hot sun. Prostitution may be illegal in Uganda but up to fifty sex workers ply their trade here, largely unmolested by the police. Their two hopes are that men will use condoms and are circumcised – but their poverty does not put them in a strong position to insist. Not surprisingly messages on HIV prevention in the fishing villages often fall on deaf ears. The fishermen live with danger; HIV is just one more risk. The consequence is that about a quarter of the population in the villages lives with HIV and among sex workers the figure is over a third.

The bleak message from Uganda is that in 2012 there were 140,000 new infections, which has propelled the overall total of people living with HIV to over 1.5 million. What makes this position doubly tragic is that a decade ago the country and President Museveni, who has been in power since 1986 when he overthrew the regime of Milton Obote, were being lauded for the way they were explicitly tackling the problem with the country's 'ABC' campaign – Abstain, Be faithful, use a Condom. In fact, Museveni's first campaign was rather different and even more challenging. It had the slogan of 'zero grazing' and was directed with some success at both men and women to persuade them to cut back on their number of sexual partners.

Officially the ABC campaign still continues, but with widely different views on its constituent parts. From the President's palace the message is that there has been far too much emphasis on the use of condoms and not enough on the A and B. In a speech (ironically on World Aids Day in 2012) Museveni criticised his own country's National Aids Commission for putting too much emphasis on condoms and circumcision, which he claimed did more harm than good. In an effort to shore up support among religious leaders in this church-going country he added, 'I think the only way to prevent Aids is through abstinence and being faithful to each other for those who are married.'

The difficulty with this argument is that, although abstinence may postpone the start of a sex life, the rest depends upon the partner. All too often the man brings infection to the relationship; a point graphically made by Canon Gideon Byamugisha, the first priest in Africa to declare himself HIV positive. 'Sixty-one per cent of all women in Africa who are HIV positive have never had sex with more than one man', he says. 'Have they waited? Yes. Have they been faithful? Yes. Are they positive? Yes.' The United States may boast about the number that have been reached with their pleas for abstinence through the President's Fund but the truth is that generalised messages of that kind are not effective and never have been.

Uganda today suffers from an agonisingly wide range of human problems. Babies are born with HIV not because the treatment does not exist to prevent an infected mother passing on her condition, but because the struggling and often inadequate health service cannot provide the prenatal care that is required. Entebbe hospital may provide a maternity unit but many other babies are born outside hospital on concrete floors covered by a blanket. Mothers get neither the advice nor the care they require and the victims are the children, who either die or inherit a lifetime illness. If the mother later dies from Aids then the unfortunate child joins the army of HIV orphans that already number over a million.

And even this is not the sum total of the avoidable misery that exists in present day Uganda. As in every country in the world there are gay men. Yet here men having sex with men is genuinely a love that dare not speak its name. Homosexuality is illegal and, unlike the law on prostitution, it is strongly enforced with enthusiastic public and media support. A few examples make the point. A writer in a *Kampala Sunday* newspaper, who clearly regarded himself as a moderate on the issue, agreed that gay men should be granted the basic rights of citizenship that 'ordinary people' enjoy but then added:

> *Where some of us start to disagree with them is when they go past demanding full legal rights in the countries they live in and actually declare or imply that there is something wrong, primitive, prejudiced and 'homophobic' about the majority of the population that finds gays odd or repulsive. A 'normal' person, that is a heterosexual, should under ordinary circumstances find the very idea of homosexuality repugnant.*

It is always difficult to find the genuine voice of the 'man in the street' but I felt we came nearest when talking with a practising Christian called Ismail. His view was that homosexuality was an illness, and that if gay people were locked up then it would prevent it from spreading. He saw it as something that could be controlled, and thought that people needed help to be 'retrained' in how to appreciate women. He added that homosexuality posed a much greater threat to the country than al Qaeda because of its perversion of people, and that Uganda should be putting more resources into tackling homosexuality than into fighting terrorism.

A much more extreme message of prejudice and hate came from a newspaper which called itself *Rolling Stone*. (It had no connection with the American magazine of that name and even less with Mick Jagger and co.) The tabloid specialised in targeting homosexuals and flourished for a few years. It published photographs of gay people, gave their addresses and incited action against them using headlines like 'MORE HOMOS' FACES EXPOSED' and 'HOMO GENERALS PLOTTED TERROR ATTACK'. It was eventually closed down after a long legal struggle – although even then the managing editor proclaimed, 'I did my job – I fought homosexuality.'

Such public and press responses reached their natural expression in a parliamentary Bill tabled in 2009 by a backbencher, David Bahati, a member of the President's NRM party, which has a large majority in the Ugandan Parliament. The bill proposed to expand the scope of the law and invented a new crime called 'aggravated homosexuality'. It set out harsher penalties upon conviction including at one stage capital punishment, although later Mr Bahati generously indicated that he was prepared to compromise with life imprisonment. Another provision was to put a duty on any citizen to report anyone they knew or suspected of being a homosexual – including family members – or face the prospect of three years' gaol in a country which does not put penal reform at the top of its priorities. It is all reminiscent of the Nazi measures against the Jews in pre-war Germany.

For several years the bill did not make its way to the floor of the House for debate thanks to the delaying tactics of the President, but no one was in any doubt of what would happen if it did. When I was in Kampala I was told by a human rights worker that if the bill was ever put to the vote 'it would be passed in ten minutes. The public are anti-gay and the politicians follow the public.' And so it proved. A few days before Christmas in 2013 the legislation was passed and two months later, in spite of all his previous hesitation, it was signed by President Museveni. A government spokesman welcomed the development 'as a measure to protect Ugandans from social deviants'.

This all leaves gay people desperately weak and wide open to exploitation. In one case (well before the latest developments) the police tipped off the media that a perfectly harmless meeting of gay and lesbian people was to take place and they intended to close 'the workshop' down. The result was that no fewer than seventy-five representatives (I will not call them journalists) of the press, radio and television turned up in force and the worst happened – pictures appeared of some of those who were attending. In another case a businessman lived with a younger man.

The police applied pressure on the younger man and persuaded him to join them in a blackmail attempt. Unless the businessman paid up the threat was that he would be taken to court on the charge that he had 'sodomised' the younger man. Knowing that the publicity would be immensely damaging, the businessman paid over the equivalent of $10,000.

Gay men, together with lesbians and transsexuals, live under constant threat of exposure. There is the risk of attack and homes being trashed. 'If they find you,' one gay activist told me, 'you will be chucked out not just from your job but also from your family home. Your mother will know that if you stay she will be ostracised and the whole household will be rejected.' Those who publicly stand up for the rights of gay people take a serious risk. In February 2013 David Cecil, a British theatre producer who had lived in Uganda for a number of years with his partner and two young children, was arrested, thrown into prison, and then put on a plane to London as 'an undesirable immigrant'. His offence was to have written and briefly staged a play which depicted a gay boss killed by his employees.

The David Kato case in 2011 showed that risk to life is not a far-fetched fear. David Kato had come out publicly and bravely as gay back in 1998. He had been one of the first members of a new group called SMUG (Sexual Minorities Uganda) and in 2010 was targeted along with other members of the group by *Rolling Stone*, which published a hundred pictures of 'Uganda's Top Homos' under the headline 'Hang them'. The magazine also included the addresses of the group. Kato and three others filed a petition to stop distribution of the magazine and this was upheld by the Supreme Court but, three months later, in the early afternoon of 26 January 2011, he was murdered in his home. There are some in Kampala who will say that this was not a homophobic crime but the kind of murder that happens too often in this poor part of the city. It is an unlikely explanation and what no one can deny is the extraordinary scene at Kato's funeral. At a service attended by family and fellow activists the preacher turned on the gays and lesbians who were present, warning of Sodom and Gomorrah. The microphone was seized by a number of activists but the villagers took the side of the preacher. Poor David Kato was only laid to rest after the former Anglican Bishop Christopher Senyonjo took over the burial. As we shall see Bishop Christopher is today a target of prejudice himself.

One inevitable result of the discrimination is that medical treatment and advice for gay men is woefully inadequate. They meet prejudice from doctors. 'Some put their religious view in front of medical ethics' said one gay man. But in constructing a health policy there is an even more basic issue. No one knows the scale of HIV among men having sex with men. Systematic research in this area has been minimal. Officials are in denial and even workers trying to reduce the spread of HIV in other areas tend to avoid the subject. As for gays and lesbians themselves, very few are going to agree to a self-reporting survey if the result is prosecution and for the same reason they are reluctant to come forward for testing. The justified fear is that the news will spread.

Yet, worldwide, men who have sex with men is one of the major at-risk populations. The one report that has been successfully completed – the Crane survey which reported in 2012 – had to contend with the arrests of some of those taking part in the survey but in the end produced results from almost 300 men. These showed that HIV prevalence at 13.4 per cent was over double the national average – and that prevalence in the over-25 age group was over 22 per cent. The survey also showed that four out of ten men had suffered homophobic abuse including exclusion, threats, insults and physical and sexual violence. A large proportion of the sample in Kampala reported buying or selling sex; many were married or cohabited and thus only too able to spread the virus further. The report warned that a lack of HIV services together with homophobia put everyone in Uganda at risk. It is a warning which has fallen on deaf ears.

So how has it come to this? Why is Uganda's antipathy to homosexuals as deeply ingrained and long established as it is? Some say that the colonial British are to blame. It was they who made homosexuality illegal and doubtless in their time were also openly contemptuous of gays and lesbians. (It needs to be repeated that it was only in 1967 that the legal ban against homosexuality was lifted in Britain itself.) But such an explanation seems heavily dated when in 2013 a Conservative-led British government can introduce equal marriage rights for gay and lesbian people. The better explanation is that in the last fifty years almost no one of real mass influence in Uganda has been courageous enough to challenge the prejudice. The President has not, Parliament has not, the press have not and, perhaps worst of all, nor have the churches.

The churches have generally played a discreditable part. Worst of all have been the American evangelists who preach as if their President did not exist, and Obama's words at his inauguration in 2013 on building an inclusive society with gays and lesbians playing an equal part had never been uttered. Their main influence dates back to March 2009 when three American evangelical Christians arrived in Kampala to plead their case, given that in the United States itself it had been widely rejected. According to the *New York Times*, their three days of meetings attracted thousands of Ugandans including police officers, teachers and national politicians. The purpose of the meetings, said their Ugandan organiser, was to show that 'the gay movement is an evil institution' whose goal is 'to defeat the marriage based society and to replace it with a culture of sexual promiscuity'.

The leader of the group was an activist called Scott Lively who was already noted for his opposition to lesbian and gay rights. Years before, in 1995, he had co-authored a book called *The Pink Swastika*. In the preface to the fourth edition in 2001 he alleged that homosexuals were 'the true inventors of Nazism and the guiding force behind many Nazi atrocities'. In March 2010 he was allowed to address members of the Ugandan Parliament and, according to his own account, urged them to fashion any new anti-homosexuality law on American laws regarding alcoholism and drug abuse.

'I cited my own pre-Christian experience being arrested for drunk driving,' he said.

> *I was given and chose the option of therapy which turned out to be one of the best decisions of my life. I also cited the policy in some US jurisdictions regarding marijuana. Criminalisation of the drug prevents its users from promoting it and discourages non-users from starting, even while the law itself is very lightly enforced, if at all.*

In other words, Lively believes homosexuality is a condition which should be medically treated and that the use of the criminal law prevents further young men being led into 'sin'. The only dispute between people who feel this way is how far the criminal law should go. Another prominent evangelical Christian is a Ugandan-born pastor called Martin Ssempa, who opposes the use of condoms to combat HIV and is a solid supporter of abstinence and fidelity; a support which earned him, at one stage, the backing of official United States aid agencies. His claim is that he leads a crusade to 'kick sodomy out of Uganda'.

Not everything, however, can be laid at the feet of the evangelists. Uganda is a church-going country and one that is also predominantly Christian – but neither the Anglicans nor the Catholics have done anything serious to defend the rights of gay men or lesbians. The basic attitude of the nine million-strong Anglican Church to homosexuality is best summarised by the former Archbishop Orombi who was leader of the Church of Uganda from 2004 to the very end of 2012. His view is that 'the younger churches of Anglican Christianity will shape what it means to be Anglican. The long season of British hegemony is over.' Among those beliefs is that homosexual practice is 'incompatible with Holy Scripture' – a view he says which is shared by the vast majority of bishops from the Global South. His reaction to the 2009 anti-homosexuality bill was that in 'streamlining' existing legislation Parliament should ensure 'proportionality' in sentencing but they should 'ensure that homosexual practice or the promotion of homosexual relations is not adopted as a human right'.

Nothing that his successor Archbishop Ntagali has said since has challenged that view – nor is he likely to do so. At the beginning of 2013, commenting on the lifting of the ban on gay clergy becoming bishops, he said, 'Our grief and sense of betrayal are beyond words.' None of this is to say that the Church (at least at the archbishop level) deliberately attacks gays and lesbians. The official attitude is that they are 'committed at all levels to offer counselling, healing and prayer for people with homosexual disorientation ... The Church is a safe place for individuals who are confused about their sexuality or struggling with sexual brokenness to seek help and healing.' Again, as so often in Uganda and other African countries, we find the assumption that gay people can be 'cured' of their affliction.

In this bleak church landscape a few figures stand out prepared to defend their fellow human beings. One of the few is Bishop Christopher Senyonjo who was expelled from the Church of Uganda for his stand on equal rights. It was an expulsion that revealed as much about those doing the expelling as it did about the man who was expelled. In a statement Archbishop Orombi said that 'the Bible is very clear that sexual intimacy is reserved for a husband and wife in lifelong heterosexual, monogamous marriage'. He added, 'For us in Uganda, pastoral care means leading people into the fully transformed life – including a transformed sexuality.' In February 2011 Bishop Christopher wrote a letter to the then Archbishop of Canterbury, Rowan Williams, in which he set out this warning.

> *When European churches failed to protect minority communities during the Second World War people were sent to the gas chambers and concentration camps … If Anglicans in one country dehumanise, persecute and imprison minorities, we must be true to the Gospel and challenge such assaults on basic human rights.*

The Church of Uganda is a long way from Archbishop Desmond Tutu who, writing in *The Lancet* in 2012, called for an end to laws which criminalised homosexual acts. He said, 'I have no doubt in the future the laws that criminalise so many forms of human love and commitment will look the way the apartheid laws do to us now – so obviously wrong.' Equally distant from the attitudes of the Church of Uganda is the Bishop of Leicester, Tim Stevens, who spoke in a rare Westminster debate on homosexuality in 2012. His view was clear – 'interference in the private sexual conduct of consenting adults is an affront to Christian values of human dignity, tolerance and equality'. Anglicanism takes pride in being a broad church, but you just wonder how even a broad church can contain such radically opposite views on such a basic question.

As for the Roman Catholic Church in Uganda (which has an estimated fourteen million members) their position is, to put it generously, equivocal. Initially it was thought that Archbishop Lwanga was alone among the different religions in opposing the 2009 anti-homosexuality bill – although when you read his words you rather wonder. The Archbishop said that the proposed law 'was not necessary considering that acts of sodomy are already condemned in the penal code'. He added, 'The Church has always asked its followers to hate the sin but love the sinner.' However, in 2012 he joined the other Ugandan bishops in a statement which said that the proposed bill was necessary as a response to 'an attack on the Bible and the institution of marriage'.

I suspect the authentic voice of the Catholic community is that of Simon Lokodo, the Minister of State for Ethics and Integrity, and a former Catholic priest. His work should be focused on anti-corruption (and goodness knows that is needed) but he told Human Rights Watch that he was someone 'empowered to uphold moral values' and that therefore he needed to address the issue of homosexuality. His view was very clear. Fighting homosexuality, he said, was a 'national priority' and those who argued for gay rights and the like were 'on a mission to destroy this country'.

It remains of course the position that the Catholic Church has a different and equally serious charge to answer: condoms. They refuse to treat condoms as either a way of birth control or, more importantly in the context of this book, as a public health provision – a way to preserve life. How many lives have been lost in Uganda and around the world by Catholic men and women following the advice of their Church?

Back in the 1980s I went to see the then Archbishop of Canterbury, Robert Runcie, and Cardinal Hume of Westminster. They were, as you can imagine, both courteous and concerned. Runcie had been dean of my college in my university days and (with substantial exaggeration) referred to me as an old pupil when we occasionally appeared on the same platform. Both promised in effect not to interfere in our campaign back in the late 1980s. That was undeniably useful at the time; an intervention from either at that moment would have seriously undermined our efforts. The trouble is that neither church seems to have moved on very far since then. The Catholic Church retains its dangerous opposition to condom use, the Anglican Church fumbles about for a position on gay people – although perhaps Archbishop Welby may just be able to lead at least one part of the Anglican community out of their present cul-de-sac.

If the churches in Uganda will not give a lead, what about the persuasive power of overseas governments and civil society organisations that finance so much of the HIV work in Uganda? They help massively in combating HIV generally and the tragic impact of it – and it is just as well they do. The contribution of the Ugandan government to fighting HIV is minuscule. The lion's share of HIV aid going to Uganda comes from the United States and the President's Fund. But even with these resources help cannot be targeted directly for the benefit of gay men and lesbians. Civil society organisations know only too well their vulnerable position and that if they become closely involved in giving help to a population that is stigmatised as criminal then the consequences for their other work could be severe. Instead, help goes into less controversial areas like the major Sunrise Scheme funded by USAID and which brings invaluable assistance and protection to around 250,000 orphans – out of a total of over a million who have been orphaned by Aids.

Most of the effort that is made directly to combat the prejudice surrounding HIV comes from groups inside the country who have defied the persecution and the risk. The outstanding example is Sexual Minorities Uganda under the leadership of Frank Mugisha, which campaigns from a small (and deliberately anonymous) compound on the outskirts of Kampala. It is a brave attempt to blunt some of the impact of official and public reaction but it reaches only a fraction of the sexual minorities they represent. Nevertheless, it shows what brave people with determination can achieve.

Of course Uganda is not remotely the only country in Africa to have laws against homosexuality. The situation varies, from countries like Nigeria where the law is enforced strictly, to countries like Kenya where the law remains on the statute book but so far is not enforced – although it still of course leaves people open to exploitation. It all poses a massive dilemma for policy makers overseas in giving aid. The United States, European governments, the foundations of Gates, Soros, Elton John and many others may be devoting massive resources to fighting HIV but they come up against policies and attitudes with which they profoundly disagree. So, what next? It is easy enough for them to stamp their feet and threaten to stop aid unless policies change. Britain has stopped direct aid to Uganda – as it happens for corruption reasons – and the direct result is that £6 million has been withdrawn from Uganda's inadequate health budget. So who do such demonstrations help? Certainly not the thousands of poor people in desperate need of help.

Nor when it comes to changing attitudes is outside influence always productive. In early 2012, the Speaker of the Ugandan Parliament went to Ottawa for an international conference, where she was roundly attacked for the policies of her country. She robustly defended them and when she returned home she was met by crowds lining the streets to give her a hero's welcome. The public reacted against what they saw as foreign efforts from outside telling them what to do. International criticism had an entirely counter-productive effect. It breathed new life into the campaign to introduce new laws on homosexuality.

The uncomfortable conclusion is that if there is to be a revolution in attitude it must be led from within. Apartheid was overcome in South Africa by the actions of brave men and women inside South Africa. The hope must be that the same will happen in countries like Uganda and that eventually it will be recognised that all that gay people are asking for is the ability to live ordinary lives not beset by stigma and discrimination. Of course, the rest of the world can help – by continuing to provide finance to treat disease, by repeating the unanswerable human rights arguments, and by their own example. There is no point in preaching equality if that just means equality for people in far off countries.

Optimistically, in time the churches will change their attitude. It seems a distant prospect but there must be men of courage who can see clearly enough the injustice of what is happening. Back in 1977 the Anglican Archbishop of Uganda, Janani Luwum, did not lack courage when he delivered a note to President Amin protesting at the regime's acts of violence. Together with the other religious leaders, he was summoned to the presidential palace. After being harangued by Amin, the other leaders were allowed to go, leaving only Archbishop Luwum – who was never seen again. The next day an announcement was made that he had been killed in a car accident. In fact he had been shot. It was a different cause but the need today is for more men like Archbishop Luwum and Bishop Christopher who are prepared to stand out for human rights. No one, however, should doubt the extent of the challenge.

I left Uganda at the end of January 2013. At the time, everyone was waiting to see whether the country would crack down even more severely on gay people. The newspaper *Rolling Stone*, which had published the names and photographs of homosexuals inciting their readers to action against them, had been closed down. But the men propounding prejudice and discrimination had not gone away. David Bahiti still lurked in the Parliament building with his anti-gay bill; the minister for ethics and integrity, Simon Lokodo, still believed that fighting homosexuality was a national priority; and the American evangelists still told gay people that they had a curable condition. As for President Museveni, he still wavered about which way to jump. Would he opt for even more repression and sign the Bill already passed by Parliament or would he try to stand out against the tide?

Twelve months later, on 25 February 2014, we received our reply. In the incongruously large state house in Entebbe and before a crowded press conference, the President signed the Bill. The result was that the promotion of homosexuality was outlawed; citizens were required to denounce to the police anyone suspected of being gay and those found guilty of repeat homosexuality could be jailed for life. Bahiti called the President's decision 'a victory for the future of our children' and Lokodo said, 'I feel very fulfilled, very elated.' Just to underline that Uganda was now intent on a new path of persecuting minorities, a national newspaper called *Red Pepper* took over where *Rolling Stone* had left off and next day published a front page story under the headline 'Exposed. Uganda's 200 top Homos'.

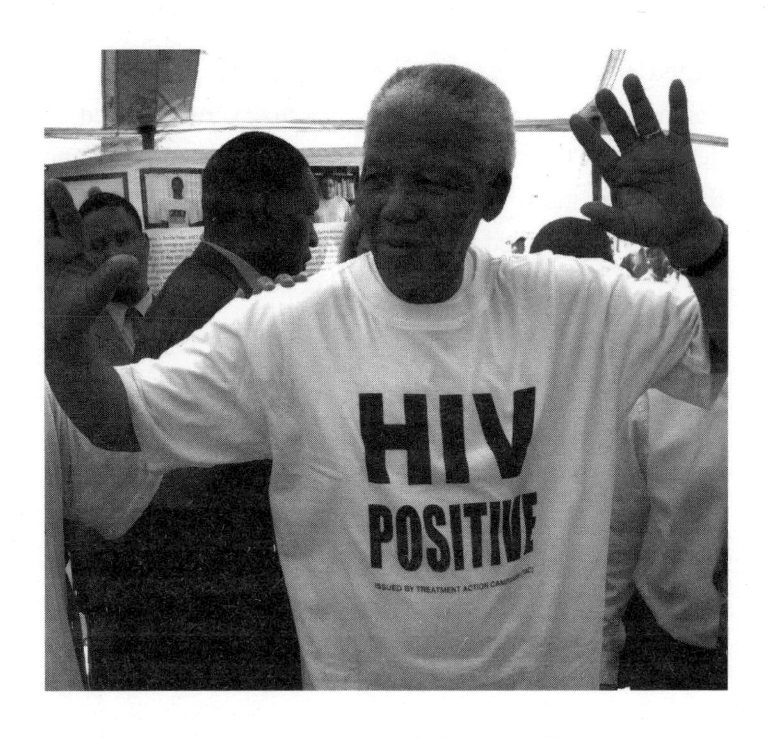

President Mandela campaigning – but his effort came only after *he had left office.*

FOUR

CAPE TOWN: IF ONLY

CAPE TOWN HAS seen the worst of times and the better times – to say it had seen the best would be an overstatement. This city, with a population of almost four million, is the parliamentary capital of South Africa, although the ministers have their offices over 800 miles away in Pretoria. The years of rebuilding South Africa after the obscenity of apartheid have been hard but successful. Today you can see the economic development. The grey towering mass of Table Mountain is part obscured by white cloud and part by the new concrete office blocks which continue to spring up. Cape Town, however, remains a city of two parts. The prosperous live in guarded mansions and neat villas and crowd the restaurants on the waterfront; the poor make do as best they can, scraping a living – if they are lucky – in jobs that the middle class reject or – if they are unlucky – confined in townships of wood and corrugated iron huts on the outskirts. HIV and Aids has been a totally unwelcome complication in the rebuilding of the nation and for over a decade it seemed to be beyond the capacity of the new ministers to control. The failure of those lost years stands as a stark warning to politicians everywhere not to delay action and, above all, not to put their 'gut' beliefs in front of objective evidence.

The political failure and human tragedy of the 1990s, now stretching into the first part of the twenty-first century, can be stated very simply: in 1983 in South Africa there was only one person recorded with Aids, a gay white man who probably contracted the virus when visiting the United States. In 1990 there were still fewer than 100,000 living with HIV. A decade later there were almost four million.

The history of the debacle is this. In the mid-1980s, when the world was waking up to the epidemic, South Africa was still in the grip of apartheid. Health care was divided by race and colour and at the centre of the apartheid policy was the promotion of private health care. In both respects this excluded the vast majority of the population. Health care was a privilege, not a public right, and the idea of a broad-based public education campaign in a country so cruelly divided was laughable. In any event, according to one activist working there at the time, 'It was simply not on the radar. That was not how they were thinking.' A favoured proposal was that those with HIV should be isolated, as TB sufferers were, which ignored the whole point about HIV that it was not infectious other than by direct blood or semen transmission. But a country that segregated people on the basis of colour could certainly do it on the basis of a little understood disease. In the face of an ineffective response the numbers infected rose, but not to the terrible heights that would make South Africa the most infected country in the world.

In 1994 apartheid fell. Nelson Mandela became President but sadly the clouds did not lift. As one health worker in Cape Town told me when I visited there in March 2013, 'The economy was the priority and making the new constitution work. Health was not the priority. If you were there at that time you might have done the same. I am not defending the inaction but you can see why.' The same point was made by a UNAIDS official in Geneva, who admitted, 'Mandela is one of my heroes but he never addressed Aids. We could have stopped it then and there had Mandela, with all his influence, said "use a condom". There was no public education.'

During those early years of the new Republic there was certainly a national plan published to combat Aids but, alas, little was done to implement it. As one provincial official lamented at the time, it 'became a neat book on the shelf'. There were not the politicians to drive the kind of campaign required, nor enough doctors and nurses in the public sector to implement it. Even when the money was available, the government misspent it, as is demonstrated in the notorious case of a 1995 play called

Sarafina II. Using funds provided by the European Union, the idea was that the play would be used to educate the public about the disease. The script was generally rated as hopeless but, above all, a play was seen as a totally inadequate response to the threat. By the end of Mandela's presidency, policy had regressed to such an extent that the government was in serious conflict with civil society organisations on two counts. The outside organisations fiercely opposed the government decision not to provide Zidovudine (AZT) to pregnant women although internationally it had become the recognised way of preventing mother-to-child HIV transmission. The second issue was almost as inflammatory. In the spring of 1999 the South African health minister, Nkosazana Dlamini-Zuma, an anti-apartheid activist who later became South Africa's minister for foreign affairs, proposed that Aids should become a notifiable disease. This would require doctors to inform immediate families and health care workers of the patient's condition. At the time she said, 'We cannot afford to be dictated to by human rights or Aids activists. It is time we treated Aids as a public health issue like TB.' The trouble with that argument is, of course, that Aids is not like TB. You can catch TB by being in close proximity to someone with the disease. It is airborne. That is not true of HIV. The result of compulsory notification for HIV is that it allows information to leak out into the local community and increases stigma when reducing it is crucial to prevention: it dissuades people from coming forward for testing when your whole aim should be to encourage them.

Of course it can be objected that at the time Nelson Mandela and the African National Congress had other massive and more important problems to tackle. Years of oppression and persecution had come to an end but there were many doubters who believed that it would be impossible to establish the new democracy. Nevertheless, from a public health point of view, the Mandela years were a disaster. New infections were taking place at a rate of 1,600 a day. A major health problem became a crisis. Like Bill Clinton, it was only several years later after he had left office (and in his case lost a son to Aids) that Mandela partly redeemed himself by joining the campaign for treatment. Perhaps the fairest verdict on his Aids record was that of the Supreme Court Judge Edwin Cameron who, in a famous speech in Durban in 2000, 'came out' as a gay man with HIV – an unprecedentedly courageous step for a sitting judge in South Africa to take. 'In 199 ways Nelson Mandela was our country's saviour,' he said. 'In the 200th way he was not.'

If the Mandela years were a public health disaster, the years that followed the end of his presidency in 1999 were a total catastrophe. In Europe and the United States, antiretroviral drugs had become widely available, but in South Africa the only sufferers able to get them were those who could afford to buy them – a point again made by Judge Cameron. His resources enabled him to buy the drugs – although eventually even he found the financial burden of paying the exorbitant drug prices from his own resources too high and had to go to friends for assistance. For the poor in the townships, there was no chance. For most South Africans, HIV remained a death sentence.

A fundamental change was desperately needed. Instead the new President, Thabo Mbeki, embarked on a deadly policy of denial. His position was that HIV did not cause Aids and at the thirteenth International Aids Conference in Durban in 2000 he promised not antiretroviral drugs but 'a better focused programme targeted at the reduction and elimination of poverty and the improvement of the nutritional standards of our people'. Translated, this meant that he believed the drugs which were saving lives in their hundreds of thousands in other parts of the world had not the same relevance in Cape Town, Johannesburg and Durban.

The theory Mbeki subscribed to was that Aids was not a result of the HIV virus but a collapse of the system brought about by extreme poverty. Antiretroviral drugs took second place to diet, and the minister of health Dr Tshabalala-Msimang (a medically qualified doctor) produced her own alternative remedies, such as the use of lemon juice, beetroot and garlic – garlic potatoes were served at one international conference. The policy did have one effect. Some people stopped buying garlic on the grounds that they did not want others to think they had HIV.

In spite of the rising death toll Mbeki stubbornly stuck to his policies and turned a blind eye to the catastrophe which had overtaken his country. Even when help was forthcoming from international donors it was either refused or only partly taken up. The government confined to a couple of pilot schemes a $72 million grant from the Global Fund to KwaZulu-Natal, although the province had one of the most severe problems in the country. In 2003, the President told the *Washington Post* that 'personally I don't know anybody who has died of Aids'.

No one can be sure how many deaths could have been avoided had this insane policy been changed. A study by Harvard University researchers suggested that on 'reasonably feasible' policies over 330,000 lives could have been saved between 2000 and 2005. The full death toll for those six years was a massive 1.76 million. If you take into account the terms of both Mandela and Mbeki the impact, particularly on women, was dire. HIV prevalence among women attending antenatal clinics stood at 7.6 per cent at the time of the first democratic elections in 1994; by 2007 it had risen almost four times to 28 per cent.

The most direct challenge to the government came from the Treatment Action Campaign formed in 1998 with the aim of achieving fair access to treatment for everyone. The campaign had its roots in Khayelitsha, a vast sprawling township of corrugated iron and wood huts just outside Cape Town itself and home to over half a million desperately poor people. If they were ever to get the treatment they needed, the campaign had to not only persuade the government but also secure a big reduction in drug prices. Inevitably this brought them into conflict with the big pharmaceutical companies, which immediately tried to block legislation to give the government powers to import or manufacture cheap versions of brand name drugs. The campaign's position was that the drug companies were 'making a killing'; the position of the drug companies was that that unless they made profits then they could not finance the research.

It is a question which still resonates today and here I declare an interest. When I was Health Secretary in the mid-1980s I introduced the 'selected list of drugs' policy in the United Kingdom. Rather than pay the branded price for drugs like tranquilisers and sleeping pills (not exactly at the cutting edge of science) I proposed we should switch to generics. It was an obvious way of putting more resources into the health service but it was fiercely opposed by the drug companies – an opposition supported, to their eternal discredit, by the British Medical Association. In New York, a dinner specially arranged for me to meet the heads of the pharmaceutical companies almost ended in a protest walk out at this 'socialist' policy. So, while I accept the argument that research needs to be financed, I am naturally sceptical about some of the claims made by the big pharmaceuticals.

In South Africa the issue came to a head in 2001 when, after a three-year legal struggle, the pharmaceutical companies (all thirty-nine of them) withdrew their case against the South African government. On the face of it, the retreat of the drug companies was a famous victory for the campaigners. In practice, the progress that followed was painfully slow. The government's policy remained broken-backed and, although the case might have been won, there were still the rules of the World Trade Organization to navigate. By 2005 less than a quarter of those who needed antiretroviral treatment were receiving it.

It was not until the autumn of 2008, when Mbeki resigned having lost the support of the African National Congress, that the real turning point came. In the reshuffle that followed the installation of an interim President, Kgalema Motlanthe, a new minister of health was appointed. Barbara Hogan was a determined politician who had joined the ANC in 1976 after the Soweto uprising and had suffered both imprisonment and ill treatment under the apartheid regime. For the first time there was a health minister who seemed to understand what HIV and Aids was all about and the importance of implementing policies that were working throughout the rest of the world. The decade of denial was at last brought to an end.

Hogan was moved inside the government when Jacob Zuma was elected President in May 2009, and the fear was that policy might weaken. But her successor at health, Aaron Motsoaledi, himself a qualified doctor, continued very much in the same vein. If there were reservations they were more about the President himself, who in 2006 had been acquitted on a charge of raping an HIV positive woman – but not before claiming in court that after intercourse with the woman he had taken a shower to 'minimise the risk of contracting the disease'.

This hardly boded well but in fact his government continued the process of reform. At the end of 2009 the Zuma Cabinet pledged to provide all HIV positive children with antiretroviral drugs. By 2010 AZT treatment was being provided for almost all HIV positive mothers with the result that mother-to-child transmission was reduced to 3.5 per cent. A public education campaign was launched – with door-to-door canvassing and advertising billboards – and KwaZulu-Natal became the first province to provide free male circumcision. The net result of the new policies is that today the number on treatment in South Africa is over two million and new infections are down from an annual figure of 640,000 in 2001 to 370,000 today. Since 2005, life expectancy has increased by six years from fifty-four to over sixty, which is claimed to be the biggest increase in life expectancy since the end of the bubonic plague – although we will skate over how exactly a comparison of that kind can be made.

Fresh initiatives have been taken throughout the country, often in cooperation with civil society organisations. If you go to Khayelitsha today you will still find the vast expanse of makeshift huts and the broken patchwork of corrugated iron roofs. But you will also find clinics where men and women wait patiently on benches from about 6.30 in the morning for treatment, which often they receive from specially trained nurses. 'We will never have enough doctors,' one of the doctors working at a clinic explained to me. The logic is to train even more nurses, particularly to work in country areas where medical facilities are sparse.

One development summarises the progress. Hospices in Khayelitska are going out of business. They are not full of HIV patients any more. Their place has been taken by 'adherence clubs' to persuade those on treatment to keep taking their drugs. The development has been pioneered by Médecins Sans Frontières, which has helped scale up treatment in Khayelitska over the last decade and has handed over almost all patients on first line antiretroviral treatment to the national health system. Instead of going to appointments at the health centre, the members of adherence clubs go to meetings (often in patients' homes) every two months for a check up and to talk to other patients. Patients can preserve their anonymity (and thus prevent rumours of infection circulating in the neighbourhood) and the result is that adherence to treatment is proved to be greater.

Keeping patients on their treatment is also part of the job of the Mothers2Mothers organisation based in Cape Town, which was formed in the dark days of 2001. They now work also in eight other African countries. They say, 'It is not enough to say we have the drugs and everything will fall into place. It doesn't. About one in three of the mothers who start prenatal treatment fall out before the birth.' Yet again one of the reasons is the stigma that surrounds the area. Mothers will choose a clinic a long way from their home to preserve their anonymity but then face the travel difficulties of actually getting there. Mothers2Mothers says that the 'stigma of HIV that is prevalent in many African communities causes women to live in fear making it difficult for them to get the care they need'.

The infection of children is no minor problem. Even now, with all the medical means at our disposal to prevent onward transmission, over 600 children are infected each day in sub-Saharan Africa. Most acquire HIV from their mothers during pregnancy, birth and breast feeding. Without medical intervention around four out of ten infants born to HIV positive mothers will contract the virus. With treatment, that number can be reduced to 2 per cent. Stigma apart, the other trouble is that health centres in sub-Saharan Africa are generally overcrowded, leaving doctors and nurses with only minutes to give proper advice. That is why Mothers2Mothers have pioneered a scheme using 'mentor' mothers, who also have HIV, to work alongside nurses and lead pregnant women through childbirth with the drugs they need. It is a long way from the garlic days of Mbeki and co.

The South African achievement is immensely important. It shows what can be achieved by political leadership when those leaders follow the medical and scientific evidence and do not go off on wild excursions of their own. It shows what can be achieved when government and civil society organisations work together. Nevertheless you are still left with an overwhelming feeling of *if only*. If only the action had been taken earlier we would not today have six million people – almost one-fifth of the adult population of South Africa – living with HIV, and if only action had been taken earlier we would not have well over a million children who have lost one or both parents due to the epidemic. Twenty years of inaction has been followed by an eventual recovery of political will – but no recovery can ever make full amends for the neglect of the past.

Nor should anyone believe that the challenges are over. South African deaths from Aids are still running at 240,000 a year. The number of young women infected by older men ('sugar daddies' as they are still called there), perhaps for the price of a mobile phone, continue to make the headlines. In the health service there are still too few doctors, with many preferring to work in the private sector or in the cities and towns and not in the country areas where providing services is most difficult. There is also the challenge of persuading the public that the denial years were the nonsense that they were. This may be the new South Africa but some of the traditional attitudes remain. There is antipathy to homosexuals; all too often women remain subservient to men, lesbian women are still raped to 'correct' them and gay men are still attacked.

The stigma around HIV still prevents men and women coming forward for testing, with the inevitable result that the disease continues to spread. One activist told me, 'Even today the level of stigma is so great that there are people who would rather die than get a test.' The fear is that the result of a test can leak out with potentially catastrophic results, particularly for women who may be ostracised by their family or assaulted by a husband or partner who in all likelihood has been responsible for transmitting the disease in the first place. A doctor in one of the townships said stigma was their biggest problem. 'People don't want to go to their local clinic for a test. They have friends and family working there. The risk is that you are pushed out of your family and you lose your job but what do I do then? That's why many say "I don't want to know".' An aid worker who had only recently arrived in Cape Town put some of this reaction down to the years of denial that have resulted in HIV being even more of a 'no go' area than in some other African countries. 'There is very high stigma particularly when you get to the rural areas. It is much higher than I expected. There is far less in Zimbabwe.'

Also inherited from the past are notorious points for infection like the mines. About half a million men work in the mines digging out gold, diamonds, platinum and coal. The men who come usually leave their wives and partners behind in the poor villages of the East Cape or over the border in countries like Lesotho and Swaziland. Unsurprisingly, sex workers, with high HIV rates, fill the need. When the miners return to their communities they take their contracted HIV (and their TB) with them – although it should be said that the big mining companies are now making great efforts to improve health care for their workers.

As for sex workers themselves, they occupy a twilight world in South Africa. One estimate puts the total number at 170,000, with perhaps 6,000 working in the Cape Town area even though prostitution is totally criminalised. It is illegal to offer sex and it is illegal to buy it. Prosecutions are rare but the legal ban means the barrier to sex workers coming forward for health checks is high, particularly as they risk abuse at the very clinics intended to help them. Their legal position makes them an easy target for exploitation. According to Maria Stacey of SWEAT, an organisation that runs a 24-hour help line, 'If they complain about rape or violence the police take no notice. Their attitude is "you are only a sex worker".' She adds an explanation about sex work which applies to many other countries around the world: 'One of the stereotypes is that they are young runaways and drug addicts. In fact only 3 per cent are under the age of eighteen. Much more typical is the poor, undereducated woman who may be a single mother and has been abandoned by the father.'

I HAVE WRITTEN about South Africa in this chapter but all the problems I have mentioned are common to sub-Saharan Africa and that certainly applies to co-infection of HIV with tuberculosis. Until very recently in the West TB was remembered as a disease of the past. We remember perhaps stories of the sanatoriums placed away from the cities and towns where there was plentiful fresh air. My own grandfather died at the time of the First World War of what was then called consumption. It was a different age. In Africa it has never been yesterday's problem. There are too many places where living or working close together provides the perfect incubator. The mines and the townships are good examples – and so too are the prisons.

In March 2013 World TB day was commemorated just outside Cape Town in the grounds of Pollsmoor high-security prison, with its double security fence set incongruously below a distant ring of surrounding mountains. A series of ministers made speeches – all good, all full of hope. 'Prison is not for vengeance but for re-education,' said one. When did you last hear a minister in the West put the point in such a way? By chance, a few days later I was in a clinic in the Khayelitsha township. On the wall was a poster which ironically promised a 'TB Transmission Guarantee' for all inmates at Pollsmoor – 220 per cent overcrowding; 23-hour lock-up in the cells and a minute amount of individual floor space.

South Africa's prison population is the biggest on the continent. It totals 160,000, including almost a third who are on remand and probably will have to wait months before coming for trial. Each month 23,000 are released but a further 25,000 take their place. No one knows exactly how many have HIV and TB but some estimates put the TB figure at over 40 per cent of the prison population. Many catch it in prison and, of course, when they are released they take it to their local community. Sometimes they have the multi-drug resistant strain of TB which is much more difficult and expensive to treat. And to be clear – you do not graduate by stages to the drug resistant kind. You can acquire it straight away if you are unlucky enough to be too near the wrong person.

You will find the same position in the prisons of Uganda, Kenya, Nigeria and in most other African nations, just as you will also find most of the issues in South Africa also raised in the other countries of sub-Saharan Africa. In Kenya (which I visited en route to Cape Town) they again have made substantial progress but 1.6 million people live with HIV. The death toll has been reduced from 130,000 in 2001 but it still runs at 60,000 a year. At the same time Kenya retains some of the old prejudices and attitudes, particularly towards homosexuals. A health minister who was brave enough to say that they should be treated like all other human beings faced calls for his resignation. An unwelcome new issue is the entry of drugs into the country, particularly affecting Nairobi and the port of Mombasa. But at least the Kenyan authorities have not set their face against all progress. They have authorised pilot schemes so that the public can be persuaded to accept the value of clean needles against all the familiar arguments. You see the political dilemma – but you also see time wasted and infection spread. In all conscience we are way beyond the time for pilot schemes: the evidence is there.

In sub-Saharan Africa as a whole there are 1,600,000 new infections a year. One reason for this extraordinary total is clear enough. In thirty-eight out of fifty-four African states, homosexuality is illegal and gay people become convenient whipping boys when political times get tough. In Nigeria for example the government has set out to make life as difficult as they can for gay men, lesbians and transgender people. In January 2014 the Nigerian President, Goodluck Jonathan, signed a law which provided for up to fourteen years in prison for gay marriage and up to ten years' imprisonment for membership of or encouragement of gay clubs, societies and other organisations. The President's spokesman said, 'This is a law that is in line with the peoples' cultural and religious inclinations. Nigerians are pleased with it.' The practical effect, apart from the cruelty aimed directly at sexual minorities, is to make it even more unlikely that gay men or women who have been infected will come forward. Would you volunteer for testing if you risked prosecution?

This leads naturally on to the very worst of all the problems facing sub-Saharan Africa. Over half of those infected with HIV do not know their condition. This is certainly serious for them personally; the later you postpone treatment the worse the prognosis is. But they are also a walking public health hazard as undiagnosed they continue to spread the virus. Nor is there any reason to believe that the position will change quickly. Too many governments regard gay men as the enemy. Too many ordinary Africans blame the woman if she contracts HIV even when she is infected by her partner. Too often the public education campaigns fall on deaf ears. How are we to win if there is this response not only in South Africa but in so many countries of the world? Surely, you think, there must be another way? How much better it would be if we could permanently prevent the disease without the campaigns on testing, without the vast and ever rising cost of drugs, without all the efforts to ensure that the treated remain on their treatment and without having to counter the prejudice, discrimination and stigma that encompasses the whole area. We come here to the biggest 'if only' of this book. *If only we had a vaccine.* Or, to be more accurate, a vaccine for HIV and a *new* vaccine for TB.

I confess to being a late convert to the vaccine cause. I remember back in the late 1980s telling press conferences that we could not expect a vaccine for at least another ten years. As the years went by with no obvious breakthrough, I put the prospect to the back of my mind. My assumption was that it was all too difficult. We would do better to concentrate on widening treatment and improving our public education messages. Two arguments persuade me that this is unlikely ever to be enough – and persuaded me also at a late stage in writing this book to join the board of the International Aids Vaccine Initiative in New York, an international non-governmental organisation that has been working on developing a vaccine since 1996.

First, I do not believe on the evidence I have seen that we are likely to cut through the prejudice that surrounds this whole area any time soon. Men who have sex with men will still fear coming forward for testing, women will still want to hide their infection, sex workers and transgender people will still be treated with contempt even inside public health systems. A vaccine will not eradicate the discrimination but it has the potential to go around it. In an ideal world, prevention of HIV would become like the prevention of polio – almost universal. In practical terms the vaccine would be used first for the very high risk groups that are the concern of all international policy. The human advantage would be immeasurable.

Second, even if none of this persuades governments struggling with financial woes, money is still an additional and very hard-nosed argument. The world is used to giving aid for medicine to cure an illness and food to stave off a famine. But with HIV it's not like that. With drugs providing management rather than a cure, the financial obligation goes on year after year. Unless something new is found the cost is in perpetuity. I wonder at times whether the world understands the size of the financial standing order it has signed.

Prevention is the most difficult issue on which to persuade governments. Treasuries are deeply sceptical of all forecasts made outside their offices. They can count the numbers but are all too sceptical on the benefits of investment. It is a dangerously blinkered policy. It does all too little to avoid future victims and future expense. Vaccine development has undoubtedly suffered from this. Over the years of the Aids epidemic governments have invested too little and the drug companies have not been prepared to take the admittedly high risk of investing in a development which may take decades to deliver or may have a big market only in low income countries where they see little chance of financial return. That again poses a problem for governments. They are used to four- or five-year election horizons. No vaccine has ever been developed in that time.

Of course the question that everyone wants answered is how long, then, will it take to develop an effective vaccine? We know that the influenza vaccine took ninety-two years to develop and typhoid over 100 years. We also know that work on a vaccine for malaria has been going on since the beginning of the twentieth century although one is finally moving towards regulatory submission. The TB vaccine, which is given to most young people, was developed over ninety years ago and has not been radically changed since, even though it is not notably effective – it certainly does not offer protection to adults in African townships. Against this, not all vaccine development has been so lengthy or so unsuccessful. Measles took only ten years to develop and Hepatitis B sixteen years; in the middle you have vaccines like the one for whooping cough which took forty-two years and polio at forty-seven years. So yes, they take time but, as Bill Gates said in London in a BBC lecture on polio, they can be spectacularly successful. In the last twenty years the polio vaccine has almost wiped out the crippling disease around the world.

Back in the 1980s immunologists thought that the development of a vaccine against HIV would be relatively easy. Sadly this was not remotely the case. In New York, Wayne Koff, chief scientific officer at the International Aids Vaccine Initiative, told me:

> *We had developed other vaccines, notably polio, but we soon found out that HIV was different. It was extremely variable on a scale we had not seen before. Whereas for most viruses there was only one or at most a handful of variants here you were looking at millions. HIV enters human cells and integrates into its genetic material, causing a lifelong infection that the human immune system cannot clear. To deal with this you need to find an Achilles heel of the virus and aim to create with a vaccine a protective immune response that out-performs mother nature.*

He added, 'We have developed vaccines for acute infections but not for a virus which lasts a lifetime. It is like a perfect storm. If you wanted to create a challenge for an immunologist this is it.'

So why, against this background, should we be optimistic today? One reason is that a vaccine trial in Thailand carried out by the US Army and the department of health in Bangkok in 2009 with 16,000 volunteers was claimed to be 31 per cent effective – initially the figure appeared even greater. A figure of 31 per cent effectiveness is not remotely high enough for licensing or use. There are some who believe that the Thailand trial is not quite as encouraging as it seems. One scientist told me, 'I would not bet my house on it.' Others, however, believe it has changed the whole position. 'It is not now a question of whether – it is a question of when,' said one Aids doctor in Europe. Hopefully we shall know the answer relatively soon with a follow-up study planned to start in 2016 in South Africa with an enhanced form of the vaccine.

There are also other reasons for optimism. There is proof of the principle that vaccination can work from studies carried out with monkeys infected with SIV. For example, when a weakened form of SIV is administered as a vaccine in monkeys, it brings down subsequent infection to undetectable levels. If similar responses could be generated by immunisation of humans, then HIV could be controlled by vaccination. It would certainly be good news if our old foes the monkeys could now have a part in producing some relief to the scourge that many believe they had a big hand in starting. And further research has produced perhaps the most hopeful signs of all in the search for the Achilles heel of HIV. These are special antibodies – known as broadly neutralising antibodies – that have the potential to protect people before exposure to the virus with the help of a vaccine.

According to Wayne Koff, who has been working on developing vaccines since the 1980s, 'In the past three or four years there has been a renaissance in HIV vaccine development with the pace of progress well exceeding the past twenty-five years.' In my view (and remember my declaration of interest) the challenge is to persuade governments to continue to invest. It is estimated that current spending throughout the world on Aids vaccine research is around about $850 million a year. That is substantially less than Britain spends on antiretroviral drugs each year. The Global Fund is precluded from spending money on research, so resources come predominantly from the National Institute of Health in Washington – just as they did when I visited them in 1987 – together with a major contribution from the Gates Foundation. Staying with the research requires an act of faith by governments and the civil society funders. So far the United States and several European governments, and organisations like the Gates Foundation, have remained steadfast, which is more than can be said for everybody.

In the autumn of 2013, British ministers received applause around the world for doubling their contribution to the Global Fund following a pledge from Andrew Mitchell, then the International Development Secretary. This decision made it all the stranger that a few weeks previously the British government cut the grant to the International Aids Vaccine Initiative from a hardly generous £8 million a year to an almost imperceptible £1 million. Although denied, the suspicion is that the reason for this volte-face by one of the first supporters of Aids vaccines is that there is no certainty that progress can be made in the five-year lifetime of a government. If this indeed is the thinking behind the policy then it is the equivalent of turning your back on an advance that could help transform the whole HIV and Aids position. We spend an extra £500 million on treatment but reduce to £1 million a year the prevention budget which holds out most chance of permanent success.

As for a TB vaccine, some think the results will come sooner than for HIV. Certainly it is the fact that the search has been continuing for much longer. The existing BCG vaccine is almost a hundred years old and, while it protects against the severe forms of TB in children such as meningitis, its reach is highly limited. It cannot be used for infants known to be suffering from HIV and has no application for adults living in the African townships. I sense here that the position could change. There are twelve vaccine candidates in clinical trials including two BCG replacements and, although the vaccine developers struggle for funds, the official position is that 'the global pipeline of TB vaccine candidates in clinical trials is more robust than at any previous period in history'.

We will have to wait and see the outcomes on vaccine development but I emphasise one point. None of this is an argument against improving our present policies to increase testing and treatment and to counter the prejudice and homophobia which scars not only Africa but a whole range of other countries as well. Vaccines are the ultimate weapons but there are no guarantees. Polio shows what can be achieved with a vaccine, but South Africa shows what can be achieved with the existing armoury. South Africa has stepped decisively back from the abyss and more than that is now taking a leadership role on HIV in Africa. Confronted with one of the biggest problems in the world they have shown just what determined action can achieve in a short few years. The tragedy is that not all African countries have been prepared to follow this African example.

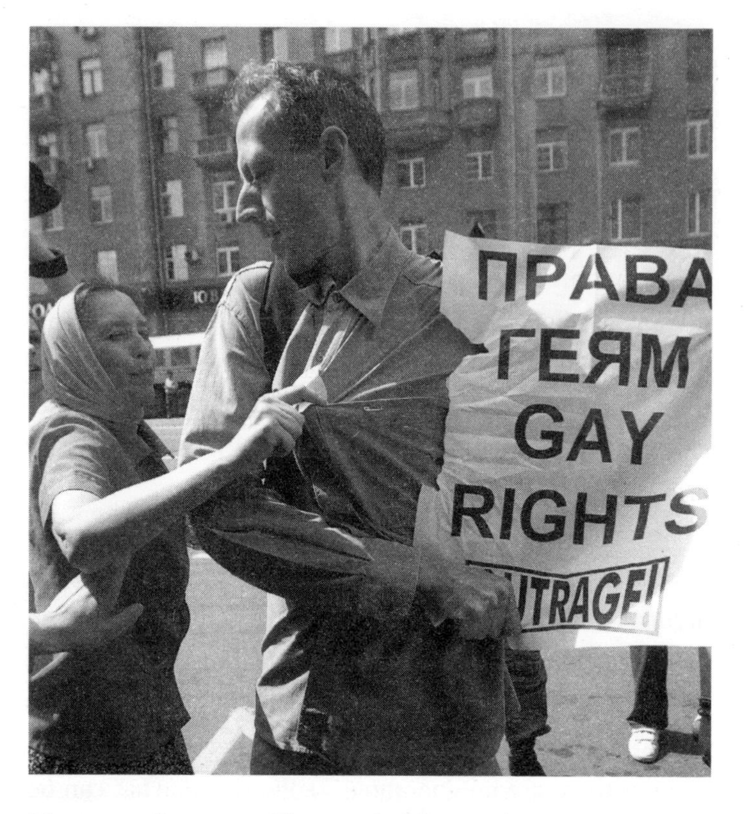

Not a popular cause. The equal rights campaigner Peter Tatchell is harangued at a demonstration in Moscow.

FIVE

MOSCOW: HEROES AND VILLAINS

BEING A NON-CONFORMIST in Moscow today is not an enviable position – as my first interview there in the summer of 2013 confirmed. It was with a campaigner on gay rights I had contacted from London. He came with an interpreter, but the interpreter wanted to start with an apology. He was standing in at the last minute. The planned interpreter had been taken into hospital. She had been part of a small, twenty-strong demonstration the day before that had protested outside the State Duma against a new law making it a criminal offence to 'promote' homosexuality. There they had been set upon by several hundred supporters of the new laws: Orthodox Christian activists and members of pro-Kremlin youth groups. Riot police had moved in and arrests had taken place, almost all of them of gay rights activists. According to the man I was interviewing, it was not the first occasion that violence had been used against the supporters of gay rights. 'It has happened two or three times before,' he said. 'Every time, our demonstrations have been broken up. Every time, people have ended up in hospital. The police do nothing about it. No one is prosecuted.'

Two weeks after I left Russia, a Gay Pride march in St Petersburg was attacked by opponents. Seven of the marchers were taken to hospital with injuries and another sixty were arrested and detained for hours in police stations. This is not a new development. The British campaigner Peter Tatchell was arrested and roughed-up four times for taking part in successive Moscow Gay Pride parades, and other stories of beatings (and worse) come from around Russia. As for the new law itself, it bans 'the propaganda of non-traditional sexual relations' to children. The untrue insinuation is, of course, that children stand in particular danger from gay men. This was certainly the excuse that President Putin used in interviews before the Winter Games in Sochi, while his Sports Minister, Vitaly Mutko, told *The Guardian* that the law was intended to protect the rights of children in the same way that they should be protected from messages promoting alcoholism or drug abuse.

In fact, the laws go beyond even the spurious defence of protecting children. They effectively make it illegal to suggest that gay relationships are equal to heterosexual ones or to distribute material on gay rights; Peter Tatchell believes that even information on safe sex may also cross the legal line. In June 2013 – twenty years after the Stalinist-era law that punished homosexuality with up to five years imprisonment was abolished – the Duma passed the new laws by a majority of 436 votes to nil. We may be in post-Soviet Russia but *glasnost* has made precious little difference. The opinion surveys show that 90 per cent of the Russian public approve the changes and that almost three quarters say that homosexuality should not be accepted by society. This is truly a homophobic country.[2]

Gays are not the only minority group who have no effective say in Russia today. If you are concerned with reducing the spread of HIV, which is what this book is all about, then the position of sex workers is crucial in almost every country. There is no easier way for the virus to be transmitted than through women and men who, by definition, have sex frequently with partners they do not know. It is not difficult to prevent transmission. The modest condom is not a revolutionary health promotion aid and, in countries that take sex work seriously, condom use among sex workers is both encouraged and is high. Not so in Russia. Rather than encourage sex workers to carry condoms, the police confiscate them.

One (admittedly small) survey conducted in St Petersburg suggested that four out of five sex workers had had condoms taken from them by the police. In other cases the very

2 Both in intent and effect the new Russian law goes way beyond the Section 28 legislation of the Thatcher years; legislation which I, for one, deeply regret.

possession of condoms has been used in court as evidence of sex work. One 24-year-old woman working in St Petersburg said that the police simply wrote in her arrest report: 'Had condoms in her possession.' The police intimidate sex workers to the point that some simply hand over their condoms once the police arrive. An obvious effect is that, rather than discouraging unprotected sex, this policy promotes it. Prostitution remains an offence in Russia although – with a hypocrisy which typifies most other countries – it is tolerated at the price of police corruption and extortion.

Yet, even when taking into account the persecution of the gay population and the exploitation of sex workers, there is no doubt which group is bottom of the Russian pile. Moscow is not like San Francisco where gay men still predominate in the total of HIV casualties. Here there is no question which is the biggest group at risk. Injecting drug users may be a small part of the problem in Western Europe, but in Russia and much of Eastern Europe they dominate the picture. Dirty needles and dirty syringes have spread the virus like wildfire to the point that Russia now has one of the fastest growing epidemics in the world.

In 2011 there were 60,000 new Russian cases of HIV; in 2012 there were over 70,000. Even in most countries of sub-Saharan Africa new cases increase but the *rate* of increase has reduced. Officially around 700,000 Russians are *registered* as living with HIV, but no one thinks that is a true measure. For a whole range of reasons many do not come forward for testing. They may fear the stigma in their town or village if the information leaks out – as it may well do. They may not want to come into contact with officialdom. They may not want to go onto the register of drug addicts and face some of the consequences that may result like the loss of a job in a country where unemployment is high. Or they may simply feel reasonably well at an early stage of the disease.

Some think a more accurate figure of the infected would probably be between 1.5 million and 2 million. More moderately, Professor Vadim Pokrovsky, the head of the Russian Federal Aids Centre, estimates the total at 1.3 million. Even that figure puts prevalence in Russia on a par with some sub-Saharan African countries once population is taken into account. According to official figures, about 20,000 Russians died from Aids and Aids-related illness in 2012 – although again the official figures are suspect and the real figure is likely to be at least double that. Where there is no dispute is in isolating the major reason for this continuing tragedy. Around 60 per cent of those living with HIV are injecting drug users. In the last few years heterosexual sex leading to HIV has become a growing part of the problem, but even this is partly because drug users have infected their partners or spouses. In contrast, the difficult-to-believe official figures claim that infection by men having sex with men is almost minimal. Given the prejudice, discrimination and now legal measures directed against them, it is hardly surprising that gay men do not volunteer information on their sexual orientation.

So why do drugs occupy such a dominating position in Russia? The official explanation is that the explosion in drug use dates from 'the American led invasion' of Afghanistan in 2001 and the vastly increased cultivation of the opium poppy that followed. One estimate is that opium production increased by no less than four times. The increased supply of heroin certainly did not help Russian efforts to stem the trade, but it is not remotely the whole story. Drug use did not start in 2001, but long before that. It was given particular impetus in the early 1990s after the collapse of the Soviet Union, the opening up of international borders and the political and social turmoil that typified the time. Unemployment and poverty added to the problems, together with young people's desire to experiment and push the boundaries of their new freedom. The number of drug users referred for the first time to drug treatment centres increased by over six times between 1990 and the start of the Afghanistan action.

Injecting is cheaper than smoking, where the user needs more heroin to produce the same effect, but heroin is not the only problem. If the price of heroin climbs or is limited because of a bad harvest then it will be diluted when sold on the street. The user needs more to get the same 'high', and the other option is to turn to cheaper, homemade alternatives which can also be more powerful. A notorious and dangerous example is *krokodil* (crocodile) named after the way it leads rapidly to scaly skin and much worse. It is made from a series of ingredients including codeine, alkaline used to clear drain blockages, petroleum from lighter fuel, and the red phosphorus from matches. All mixed and injected. To curb its use the authorities have now stopped the over-the-counter sale of codeine, but no one doubts that addicts will find other ingredients and other products.

On the face of it, Russia would seem an open and shut case for harm-reduction policies. The availability of clean needles and syringes would cut off the transmission route of HIV among injecting drug users; the controlled supply of methadone would take drug users off injecting and offer the potential of taking them off drugs altogether. Around the world many other countries, quite apart from Britain, have established beyond any reasonable doubt that clean needles, syringes and methadone is a policy that works and can all but eliminate this method of transmission.

You might think that you don't need a crystal ball to predict the results of harm-reduction policies when the evidence is so clear. In Russia, however, such policies are rejected out of hand. Dr Sergey Muraviev from the Ministry of Health says: 'Russia is against methadone treatment. Drug users can't be treated with drugs. Our aim is to take people off drugs altogether. Methadone leads to the death of patients.' His words are echoed by Dr Gennady Onischenko, who until very recently was the Chief State Sanitary Physician and who, in spite of this rather strange title (at least to British eyes), had a wide responsibility for public health. He is now an adviser to the Prime Minister, Dmitry Medvedev. His opposition to methadone is absolute.

'There is not enough evidence it works,' he says, echoing the words of the Edinburgh police thirty years ago. 'If we make drugs legal then it will damage the overall position.' We should not be totally surprised at the Russian approach today. Throughout the twentieth century there was an unequal battle between the traditional psychiatrists, called narcologists, who specialised in alcoholism and drug dependency and believed that addiction was a mental illness best dealt with in an asylum or a labour colony, and a few physicians who supported maintenance as a means to a more or less normal life. The story is set out by a Russian historian, Dr Alisher Latypov, who says that the characteristic response of Communist officialdom to both alcoholism and drug dependence was to back the traditional psychiatrists. The dependent were 'morally depraved' and 'degenerate' and certainly not the kind of people who should be treated with kid gloves. In the 1920s the main debate was how quickly they could be forced off their addiction – abruptly, rapidly (within one to two weeks) or gradually (one to two months). In Moscow the abrupt method held sway. Among the supporting theories put forward to justify the hard line was that compulsory work inside a labour colony was an effective form of therapy, and had the added advantage that it could be organised on a self-supporting basis without placing a financial burden on the state. Even more optimistically, it was hoped that the Communist state would provide its own inherent solution by establishing human rights and ending the economic exploitation which was common to capitalism, which the Soviets blamed for drug addiction.

There were occasional breaks in this line of repression. For six years at the beginning of the 1930s there was in effect a maintenance programme in what was then Leningrad (now, after a referendum, back to its old name of St Petersburg). Morphine and heroin addicts were maintained on opiates (at a reduced level) on the basis that much of their inherent problem was their constant concern about the cost of obtaining the drugs and the inevitability of 'an underground life'. The authors of the scheme claimed significant success, including one patient whose case has a total resonance today. He had used morphine and heroin for eighteen years and had been treated unsuccessfully by narcologists three times. He was unemployed and his whole body was covered with sores. Very soon after enrolling on the maintenance programme he found a job and switched from using drugs intravenously to an oral solution of heroin. Other cases were equally successful but then the programme was caught up in a wave of Stalinist repression which could not tolerate the idea of the drug dependent being treated with such 'generosity'.

A more difficult question for the authorities was what to do with the 'hero addicts'. These were the men wounded fighting in the Second World War and who became dependent on morphine. The supply of opium was crucial to ease their pain. During the war all the harvest from the Kyrgyz poppy fields had to go to the front and anyone trying to divert the harvest was shot on the spot. Once the war was over the soldiers who had become addicts could hardly be abandoned. Maintenance treatment was continued but, as the narcologists made clear, it was for the 'soldier heroes', not the villains and degenerates who began to dominate the addiction figures as the years went by. Today there is no doubt what the policy is: no clean needles, no syringes and, most of all, no methadone.

The theory that you cannot use narcotics to maintain and hopefully withdraw the users from their addiction prevails over alternative claims put forward by the few campaigners brave enough to say that the Russian government's policy is not only a nonsense, but is also responsible for thousands of unnecessary deaths. In the words of one Russian I met who was working in the field, 'They persist in looking on drug users as criminals not patients. Their one and only goal is to force them onto abstinence.' Another told me: 'The official attitude is that there should not be an easy way to get off drugs.' The Moscow-based Andrey Rylkov Foundation agrees, saying 'Russian drug treatment standards are outdated and based on repressive approaches that were in practice during Soviet times.' The foundation is a grassroots organisation established in 2009 to advocate for humane drug policies, including opioid-substitute treatments like methadone. They quote the view of one official who characterised the official approach as 'you suffer – and next time you won't do anything bad'.

The sanctioned treatment is one of withdrawal from opioids altogether. In Moscow I asked a senior doctor how this was organised. He rather wearily mopped his brow. There were, he said, a hundred different programmes. At its best, treatment might consist of three to twelve days of detoxification followed by several months of outpatient supervision or treatment in a rehabilitation centre. The gaping hole in the policy is this: there is no shortage of state-run detoxification centres but, by themselves, they will rarely lead to a drug-free life. So much depends upon rehabilitation and the follow up. Here the facilities do not remotely match the demand, with the effect that the overwhelming majority relapse back into drug taking. 'The doctors see them coming back and coming back,' said one researcher. 'They are clean for twenty days and then go back to the same environment and the same dealers.'

In 2006 one rare independent survey, of almost 1,000 injecting drug users in ten Russian regions, by the Penza Anti Aids Foundation showed that almost 60 per cent of those who had made use of the state treatment system had gone back to using drugs within a month of finishing their treatment course. More than 90 per cent had relapsed within a year. This finding was confirmed by the Russian Federal Drug Control Agency which in a 2009 report said that over 90 per cent of drug treatment patients resumed the use of illegal drugs within a year.

Another survey carried out with injecting drug users in Volgograd and Barnaul showed that, although most users received detoxification, only a third received any kind of rehabilitation. One of the chief fears which prevented drug users coming forward was the effect that this could have on their employment prospects. Those who do come forward are registered as drug users by the local drug treatment service, and the fear is that registration becomes 'a stamp on the forehead' which is taken as a sign of degeneracy by both employers and the police. The survey said: 'Drug users have little trust in the treatment system, perceive the system to be as much a hindrance as a help, and associate treatment with high failure rates, short remissions and continuing drug use.'

One of the main authors of the report, Natalia Bobrova, summarised the position for me:

> *The main issue within the governmental treatment programmes is the sole focus on detoxification and the lack of good rehabilitation programmes. There is a lack of funding and training and a lack of highly qualified specialists. It leads drug users to turn to obscure private treatments like City Without Drugs and traditional healers.*

The opposite view is put by Yevgeny Roizman, a co-founder of City Without Drugs, who in the autumn of 2013 was elected mayor of Russia's fourth largest city, Yekaterinburg, on the basis of his outspoken views. A 2012 *New York Times* article described the City Without Drugs approach as 'kidnap and cold turkey', quoting one worker as saying, 'We know we are skirting the edge of the law. We lock people up, but mostly we have a written request from their family. The police couldn't do this, because it's against the law.' Roizman himself explained the principle of his approach to the *New York Times*. 'The most important thing is to force them to quit and keep them clean a certain time so that the system cleans itself out. If they behave they can go home.'

Such a defence brings another complaint about the Russian treatment system. Not only is it ineffective, the methods used in the usually unsuccessful attempts to force the dependent off drugs can be brutal. The stories are difficult to substantiate but they come thick and fast – particularly from inside the private sector. There are stories of drug users being handcuffed to their bed frames, undergoing electric shocks and even of mock burials where the patient is put in a coffin and left in the ground for fifteen minutes. The idea of this last form of 'treatment', I was told, was to deliver 'such a profound shock to the drug user that he will reconsider the whole experience of his life'.

More substantiated are two cases quoted in a 2011 report put together by a number of civil society organisations led by the Andrey Rylkov Foundation. One 28-year-old drug user recounted his experience in a state-run clinic:

When I came to the clinic I was prescribed sleeping pills and pain killers but I was feeling really very bad. I asked nurses to give me more medication but instead the nurse called the clinic's ward assistants and I was tied to the bed for twenty-four hours. After twenty-eight hours they untied me but I had developed deep lesions and wounds in my legs. The skin was gone – baring the tissue as under the influence of tranquilisers I did not quite understand what was going on ... Many of my acquaintances encountered this kind of treatment practice. Many of them are already dead.

The second case concerned a private rehabilitation centre. Such centres have sometimes been given carte blanche by relatives who have referred the patient, and conditions can be even worse. A 31-year-old patient described the deliberately violent methods used, particularly against new entrants to the rehabilitation centre who are considered the most likely to be deterred. He described how men were taken to a separate room, stripped to their underclothes and then effectively beaten up by three of the staff with clubs and shovels. 'They were asked: "So are you going to inject drugs again? Will you?" Everyone shouts – "No, I will not. I am not going to use drugs any more. I swear. Just stop the flogging. Don't flog me any more please."'

The International Network of People Who Use Drugs says, 'In Russia today we are bearing witness to one of the biggest avoidable catastrophes in the history of HIV.' Human Rights Watch says that the treatment offered at drug treatment clinics in Russia is 'so poor as to constitute a violation of the right to health'. And so the criticism goes on. There is too much agreement between them all to write it off as some plot from outside to discredit Russia. The Russian authorities seem to be intent on doing that for themselves.

There remains then their argument that methadone treatment simply substitutes one drug for another and brings no long-term benefit. It is an argument that again is rejected by virtually all medical authorities including the World Health Organization and UNAIDS. Methadone is taken orally and doses are given once a day. The very least that it will achieve is to take men and women off injecting and virtually close down this route to HIV and Aids – a massive gain in itself. It is true that methadone is an opioid like heroin, but it works in an entirely different way. It lasts longer in the body and takes away the craving for heroin. The enormous advantage to those who move to methadone is that they can often hold down a job, reunite with their families, and avoid the constant pull of the drugs underworld.

The real complaint against methadone is that it maintains the drug user but it does not automatically lead to a drug-free life. This argument marks a fundamental divide on what the purpose of treatment should be. Politicians (and not just in Russia) hanker for a cure-all: an end to drug dependence and total abstinence. But most physicians would say that this will often not be possible. As one British report says, 'Recovery is an individual process or journey rather than a pre-determined destination.' Difficult as it may be for some to accept, the truth is that stabilising a drug user on methadone may be as far as you can get. Nor need that be regarded as failure. It enables the man or woman to live an otherwise normal life and to hold down a job. It also preserves them from the much greater danger of injecting and shared needles – and allows them to avoid not only heroin but the highly damaging drugs cooked at home.

None of this is likely to persuade the Russian authorities any time soon to change their policy, in spite of all the signs of its failure. According to one campaigner I met during my visit to Moscow, the police and the special 40,000-strong federal drug control service pursue a policy not so much of zero tolerance to drugs as 'zero tolerance to the drug user'. The drug users are easy meat for the police. It is easier to arrest them than the much more dangerous pushers or to break up the criminal gangs. In one case, a well-known addict was followed to his flat by a policeman who then waited for two hours outside on the street. When the addict re-emerged he was arrested, taken to the local station, beaten and left for thirty-two hours in a cell. 'The trouble is that the police officers don't feel they are doing anything wrong,' my informant said. 'They are repairing an omission in the legal process.'

Corruption in this process is inevitable and it is not always the corruption of organised crime. A notorious case was that of Taisiya Osipova, an opposition activist, who in 2012 was sentenced to eight years' imprisonment for *possessing* heroin – and the sentence was twice as long as the prosecutors had sought. The overwhelming number of drug cases that go to trial in Russia (over 90 per cent) result in convictions, and this was no exception. No one suggested that she was a trafficker and all the evidence was that the drugs had been planted on her by the police.

Prison also brings into play the two other killer diseases closely linked with Aids. The first is tuberculosis (as in South Africa), which is often the final cause of death for an Aids patient whose immune system has been destroyed. The other is Hepatitis C, which is caused by shared needles and eventually leads to cirrhosis of the liver. The problems caused are not unique to Russia – they too are worldwide. Nevertheless an overcrowded prison is the perfect incubator for TB and Russia has a massive prison population of over 900,000. As for Hepatitis C, it flourishes when shared needles are the chief way of injecting.

While Russia continues to defend its reactionary approach, elsewhere in the world drug policy is under a new scrutiny. As the years have gone by, we have all heard claims for a single solution to eradicate drug use or listened to a variety of optimistic claims. I remember being in Tehran in the 1960s at an Interpol conference where police chiefs believed the solution was to substitute sunflower for the opium poppy in Afghanistan. That failed, as did the much more recent attempt to persuade opium farmers to grow wheat and guarantee the market price. Some say that the only effect of that was to increase the supply of fertiliser, which was an all too ready ingredient for homemade bombs! As for more bellicose slogans, I remember being given a T-shirt by the Drug Enforcement Agency in the United States embroidered with the words 'It's not over until we win'. That was over twenty years ago, and I fear the 'war on drugs' has claimed no victory.

In the days before I arrived in Moscow I was at a harm-reduction conference in Vilnius, the capital of Lithuania, a country once a part of the old Soviet Union. There Michel Kazatchkine, the former director of the Global Fund to Fight Aids, succinctly set out the case for reform. Present policies on drugs had failed, he said. 'No other social policy has attracted such support from the politicians in spite of all the evidence that it is ineffective. We stick to the repressive policies even though there is so little evidence of progress.' And why? There is a political attraction in the rhetoric of 'the war against drugs' and 'being tough'. A few days after I returned from Moscow I heard a strikingly similar message at Westminster from the Colombian ambassador in London who, speaking on behalf of his government, used almost the same words to support change in his country; Columbia of course has been long regarded as almost a by-word for illicit drugs. Another straw in the wind came a few months later when Gallup in the United States reported that, for the first time in history, a majority of the population supported the legalisation of marijuana.

Michel Kazatchkine is right. We have been mesmerised by the rhetoric and with the thought that with one last push the problem will be over. Now, in the second decade of the twenty-first century and for the first time I can remember, there is a serious movement for change. Politicians are beginning to search for solutions rather than phrases which might go down well with the public. It is not happening everywhere, but there is a movement. Needless to say it is a movement in which the Russians are playing no part. There, the old and unsuccessful policies will continue to be pursued; the war on drugs has become, in the words of the prominent Russian politician, Boris Gryzlov, 'a *total* war on drugs'.

As if all this was not bad enough, almost nothing effective is done to warn the Russian public of the dangers of HIV. There are none of the poster campaigns that have been mounted in North America and Britain. Television stations refuse to take advertisements which might offend their viewers. The government devotes a minute part of the health budget to prevention. While this is true of other countries, most of these nations – certainly in the West – do not have a problem of the same scale. The doctors I spoke to in Russia were united in saying that there was a false complacence about the Russian position; that public information was seriously inadequate while sex education in schools could be non-existent.

So are there, then, no bright spots in the dark Russian landscape? There are a few. Antiretroviral treatment in Russia is not remotely adequate, but it is provided. About 120,000 HIV patients currently receive treatment, but that should be compared with the mountainous need. There are promises (budget pressures permitting) that the number of people receiving treatment will increase by 2015. A more certain positive trend is the substantial reduction in mother-to-baby transmission that has been achieved, with the result that many fewer babies today are born with HIV, and at a hospital near St Petersburg there is an example of what can be done for those children who have been unlucky enough to inherit or acquire the virus.

A short drive from the ornate gold of the Winter Palace and the crowds visiting the rooms lined with old masters in the Hermitage there is a hospital built for the poor at the time of Tsar Alexander II. The hospital has developed over the years, surviving revolutions and wars – including the siege of Leningrad, when over 600,000 Russians perished in one of the bravest actions of resistance during the Second World War. The hospital came to treat HIV in the late 1980s when almost 300 children were infected by used syringes, which rapidly spread the virus. This was at a time before antiretroviral drugs and also a time of stigma and ignorance. There was public fear that in some way HIV was infectious merely through touch or proximity. The little children who came to the hospital did not go to local nursery schools because, in the words of the chief medical officer, Professor E. E. Voronin, 'the nursery schools would not have them'. A petition signed by 2,500 local people was sent to President Yeltsin calling for the clinic to be closed and indeed it was, but for only twenty-four hours, after which wiser heads prevailed.

Today, the hospital operates in calmer but still difficult waters. The HIV orphans are potentially the most heart rending of the HIV casualties. In truth, many of the children are not there because of the deaths of their mothers, but because they have been abandoned by drug-dependent parents. 'Each of them dreams of a family,' says Professor Voronin. 'Many of the children think that their mothers lost them. Our aim is to give the children a future. The medical treatment is only part of that.'

The older children go to school locally – although their condition remains secret – while the younger ones have their own nursery and a dedicated staff try to repair some of the damage that has already been done. Professor Voronin says that in one case a three-year-old girl had been left for months in isolation and when she came to the clinic her face was like a mask. There were no smiles and no reactions. In another case, a child had been sent to an institution for invalids.

Much of this can be put right by the devoted care the children receive at the hospital. Even more hopefully, an increasing number of children are being adopted. Over half of the HIV orphans realise their ambition of a family. The easiest to place are the very young girls of two or three, the most difficult are the children of school age – although that is the common experience of all adoption agencies. Until recently, one possibility was for children to be adopted outside Russia. The nurses all remember a boy adopted by an American couple and who developed into what is regarded in St Petersburg as a typical American teenager. That route has now been closed by the Putin government, which has decreed that there should be no more foreign adoptions – a particularly malevolent restriction when dealing with still hard-to-place children with HIV. Doubtless, the St Petersburg hospital will overcome this obstacle, as they have other obstacles over the past 135 years. What is decidedly less sure is whether Russia will develop successful policies to combat injecting drug use and prevent the HIV infection being spread.

Beyond these small pools of light, the Russian picture remains very dark. The numbers of the infected continue to rise while the government remains hostile to gay people, drug users and sex workers – exactly the groups that can most easily spread the virus. Almost all the signs that have come from the Kremlin have been unhelpful to the cause of reducing HIV. As well as the anti-gay bill that was passed in June 2013, other pieces of legislation have the same baleful impact. Another bill bans so-called foreign agents. USAID, which had provided invaluable support, has already fallen into this category. In the case of USAID you could sympathise perhaps with the Russian doctor who asked me, 'What would you say if the Americans put a development agency in the middle of London?' But that does not explain it all. The inevitable result has been that any non-government organisations with any kind of overseas backing fear that the axe will next fall on them – as I saw for myself. In the autumn of 2012 I had been urged by a particular charity to visit them. My visit had to be postponed for six months and in that time their attitude changed. They suddenly needed to know whether I could set out the purpose of my trip and what questions I would be asking. I do not blame the organisation. It simply shows the nervousness that has been engendered among good people who only want to help.

My hope had been to put some of these points to the then chief physician (now prime ministerial adviser) Dr Onischenko, who is reputed also to be close to President Putin. In the event it turned out to be one of the most bizarre interviews I carried out for this book. He had three major points. His first was to ask whether I was writing a work of fiction or non-fiction. It was a point that I (mistakenly) treated as something of a joke. In fact I think he was serious. It was another way of asking whether I was going to tell the truth or make up lies about the position in Russia. This was allied to his second point. Put bluntly, he wanted to know what God-given right had a Conservative politician from Britain to sit in judgement?

Perhaps I could answer that as doubtless others – particularly some of the ministers and officials who I interviewed – had something of the same reaction. This is a book by a politician who used to be a journalist and who regards the standard of fair reporting I was required to meet on the London *Times* of the 1960s as still being the standard to follow. It is for others to judge whether the fact that I am a Conservative politician has any particular relevance.

I certainly do not deny a political intent. Researchers may research, writers may write, but when it comes down to it you need politicians to run with the policies. The truth is that around the world there are policies being pursued which are adding to the already mountainous toll of the dead from Aids. If they can be persuaded to change tack or be helped in what privately they want to do in any event then I would regard that as entirely worthwhile. I have no 'God-given' right, but if this little book helps save just one life I will be satisfied. Which brings me back to Dr Onischenko.

His third point was his most complacent and held most danger. The Russian public, he said, were well satisfied with how the government was responding to HIV although, as we have seen, public information is sparse. In his view viruses and diseases came and went. There were others which would afflict us in the future. We had seen off smallpox, cholera and legionella, and we would see off HIV as well. He had no doubt of that. The trouble – the literally fatal flaw – with this argument is: what happens in the meantime? No one realistically believes that a cure is likely to be available overnight or that it could be administered globally and instantaneously even if it was. There are measures that can be taken *now* to enable people to live successfully with HIV but that is of no comfort if the measures are ignored or only partially implemented.

The truth is that this is all a blue print for inaction. Apart from the promise (budget considerations permitting) to increase antiretroviral treatment nothing much will change in Russia. The drug dependent will continue to become infected. Gay people will continue to be a target for discrimination. Sex workers will continue to be exploited. The public will not be warned of the dangers of Aids – and men, women and children will continue to die from this neglect.

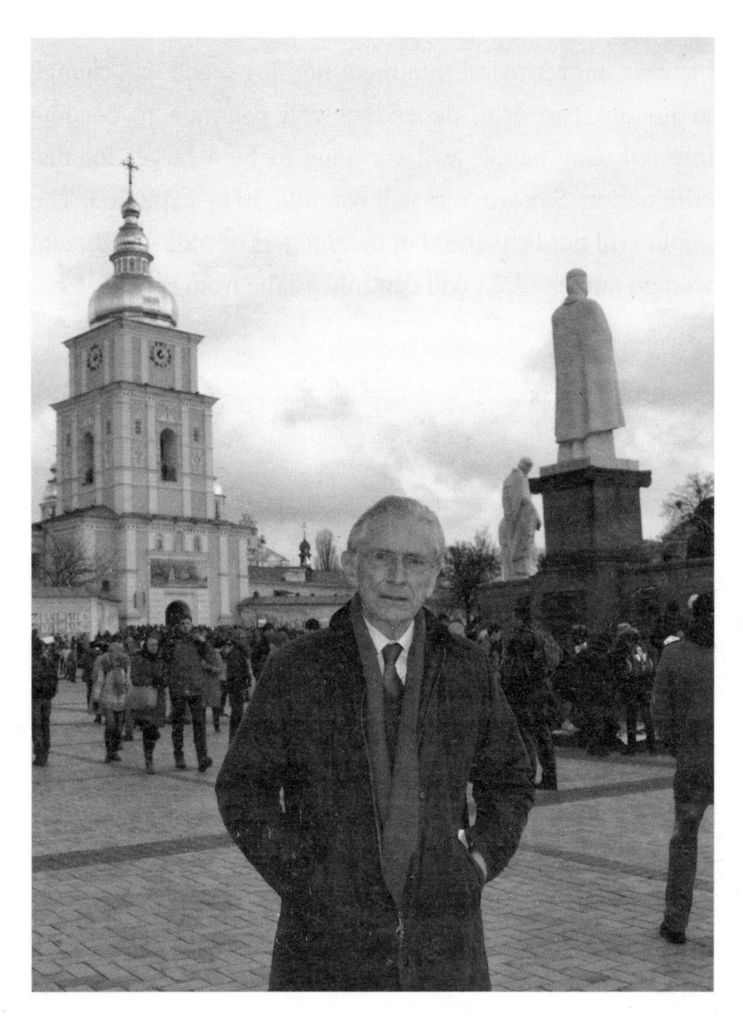

Norman Fowler in St Michael's Square in December 2013, at the start of the Kiev 'revolution' which led to a series of unforeseen consequences.

SIX

KIEV: A NEW START FOR UKRAINE?

IT IS ALMOST ten o'clock at night in Independence Square in Kiev. The temperature has fallen to below zero and there are the first flakes of snow. In the square the blue and yellow flags of Ukraine fly in the stiff breeze, side by side with the dark blue flags of the European Union. A great shout goes up: 'Honour to Ukraine. Honour to our heroes.' In spite of the bitter cold the square is crowded with several thousand demonstrators keen to support closer links with Western Europe and opposed to the government, which has just retreated from going down that path in the face of Russian threats. Smoke fills the air from the wood burning in large canisters. In the crowd there are many young students but many others who are much older – including a disabled man with an EU sticker taped to his mobility vehicle. The atmosphere is relaxed, almost carnival-like. A young man enthusiastically shakes my hand when he discovers I come from London. There is no hint of violence – not, that is, until six hours after I had left.

At four o'clock in the morning of Saturday 30 November 2013, the dark-coated riot police lining one side of the square, but not interfering, suddenly advanced in a violent change of tactics. Most of the television companies had stopped transmitting; most of the photographers had given up for the night. The demonstrators who remained were beaten and forced back, and the square cleared and closed. The direct result was that the next night a far bigger crowd gathered in a different square only a quarter of mile away as passing cars hooted their support. It was the first night of the Kiev revolution which led to the fall of the government of President Yanukovych and the unforeseen intervention of Russia in Crimea.

Amidst this political turmoil the question for gays and lesbians in Kiev was whether this movement for change would include them or whether their position would be ignored and they would be no better off than before. Homosexuality has been decriminalised since the collapse of the Soviet Union in 1991, but that does not mean that the cause of equal rights is embraced even by the political reformers. Public hostility to homosexuality is deeply ingrained – so much so that it is a political card to play when the conditions are right. In the national debate running up to the 2013 trade talks in Vilnius (which were the original cause of the Kiev demonstrations) Russian-financed advertisements appeared on the Kiev metro threatening what the consequences of closer links with the EU would be. One promised higher prices, another threatened unemployment while a third showed two men walking hand in hand. The message was crude and clear: go West and you will get free love and gay marriage.

Messages like this are most enthusiastically and inevitably supported by the biggest church in Ukraine, the Russian Orthodox Church. But most of the other churches in this country of many religions are no better. The Ukrainian Orthodox Church, formed amidst much religious controversy at the time of independence, does not share the political views of its Moscow counterpart. When the demonstrators were attacked by the police in Independence Square, the wounded and frightened were given shelter in the St Michael's Church – once destroyed by Stalin but since rebuilt. The head of the Church, Patriarch Filaret, is openly in favour of not only closer links with the West but also membership of the European Union. That does not mean the Church intends to campaign for equal rights for sexual minorities or anything close to it – before the first gay pride march in Kiev, the Patriarch warned that people supporting gay rights would be cursed. Away from the Orthodox churches, Archbishop Sviatoslav Shevchuk of the Ukrainian Catholic Church rebuffed a suggestion that he was a liberal on homosexuality. In an interview in 2012 he said that homosexuals deserved support and pastoral care but that 'in accordance with the teaching of the Church, homosexual behaviour is a grave sin which calls to Heaven for vengeance'.

It was the first gay pride march here in May 2013 which brought many of these feelings to a head. The organisers had struggled hard to avoid a ban and eventually about a hundred brave souls took to the streets. There they were met by protesters five times their number. A number of protesters chanted 'Ukraine is not America: Kiev is not Sodom'. A group of nuns carried religious icons while a photographer captured a symbolic picture of a bearded priest brandishing a chair against the sexual interlopers. The basic Christian belief of 'good will to all men' was put to one side so that the battle against 'evil' could be pursued.

An even starker example of the religious prejudice that exists in Ukraine was the case of the clinic set cheek by jowl, but separate from, the famous Russian Orthodox Lavra Monastery with its crowning gold globe that can be seen for miles around. There had been a clinic on this site since the First World War and since 1947 it had been the national centre for infectious diseases. Twenty years ago it took on responsibility for HIV and Aids. This proved to be a fatal error. The monks next door protested and as the years went by pressed for the clinic to be moved away. As one said only too revealingly, 'It is unpleasant to live next door to people who have sinned all their lives and got all the diseases you can get.'

In spite of international and national pressure, and a number of patients who handcuffed themselves to their beds, the doctors and nurses were moved out in the autumn of 2013. One of the last patients to be ejected said that representatives from the monastery came in to tell him that it was now under their control. 'They were not interested in what I was saying about the need for treatment,' he told me, 'just possession.' The clinic now stands in darkness; the curtains have been taken down and the wards and consulting rooms are empty. The authorities will point to the new clinic which has been built well away from the monks of the Lavra Monastery. But the truth is that, however good the new clinic proves to be, the motivation for the move was not to provide better facilities for those living with HIV, but to appease the monks. The government caved into the pressure of the Church.

Under the presidency of Yanukovych, it was not gays walking hand in hand that the Ukraine population needed to be wary of, but the government and Church in firm embrace. The point was rammed home in a postscript to the beginning of the Independence Square demonstrations. By the end of the first week of protest thousands upon thousands had taken to the streets and were proving far too quick-witted for the police and the authorities generally. When one square was closed they moved to another; when all squares were banned they moved to a park and in the end they just moved back to where they had started. Fighting to catch up, the government badly needed a counter-demonstration to be organised. It was much smaller – although doubtless it would have been bigger in one of the cities in the east of the country – but where was the starting point of the demonstration? It was, of course, the Lavra Monastery.

For myself, I remain as utterly puzzled as I did back in 1986 by this kind of antipathy. So why does it happen in a European country, with a population of forty-seven million in a land area about the size of France, and only a short air journey from London and Paris? Why is there this hatred of gays, lesbians, drug users and the other minorities? After all, the whole population is not devoutly religious. Stalin and his successors did all they could to stamp out organised religion. In Africa and India the excuses and explanations for homophobia go back to British colonial rule and the repressive laws passed then. That can hardly be the reason in Ukraine. The British seem to be one of the few invaders that this country has avoided. Anna Reid, in her brilliant book *Borderland*, describes the nation's troubled history. She describes how Ukraine was split between Russia and Poland from the mid-seventeenth century to the end of the eighteenth, between Russia and Austria through the nineteenth, and between Russia, Poland and Czechoslovakia between the two world wars. Until the Soviet Union collapsed in 1991, it had never been an independent state. Rival armies fought over it; powerful nations occupied the land and committed the most appalling crimes against the people living there. In particular there was the Soviet-induced famine of the early 1930s, when an estimated five million men, women and children were deliberately starved to death in the name of 'collectivisation'. It was one of the most under-reported human tragedies of the twentieth century.

Like other countries in Eastern Europe, Ukraine persecuted its minorities, and in particular the Jews. Long before the horrors of the holocaust, Ukraine had its pogroms. The Tsarist rulers found it useful to have convenient scapegoats and used anti-Semitism to take attention away from local dissent. Perhaps what we saw in Kiev was a variation of that. For any government or political party it is useful to have a convenient set of 'villains' to blame to take attention away from their own failings. In the West it is currently immigrants; here homosexuals and drug addicts have been made the bogey-men. In Ukraine (as in Russia) their vilification provides a convenient distraction from the real national evil – which was and is official and private corruption.

As for the public it is possible that, without the Jews to persecute, homosexuals and transgender people simply moved up the intolerance scale. Perhaps those who have been persecuted themselves (and no one can doubt what Ukraine has had to bear) look for someone else to persecute. Or perhaps, as one young Ukrainian suggested to me, it is a legacy of Soviet rule. 'Soviet society was for the strong and the well-performing,' he said. 'Gays were regarded as weak.'

Whatever the explanation, this is a country where prejudice and discrimination have permeated all parts and where minorities have been treated with contempt – and worse. When I was first in Kiev in 2012, I held a meeting with organisations representing drug users, men who have sex with men and sex workers. I listened to a long list of complaints of police harassment and corruption backed by courts who would invariably accept the police story. At first I was inclined to think that the claims were being embellished until a charity worker intervened. 'I can confirm all they say,' he interjected quietly. 'I was in the police for thirteen years. That's why I left.' A small example of the public view came when I was taken to a tiny drugs clinic tucked away in the corner of a hospital on the outskirts of Kiev and surrounded by the bleak concrete blocks of flats so loved by Soviet architects. 'Be very careful with your car,' we were told. 'They are dangerous people you are visiting.' The speaker was a *nurse* from another part of the hospital. Even among those receiving the (albeit inadequate) antiretroviral treatment there is discrimination. Your chances of receiving treatment are seriously reduced if you are drug user – some say less than a fifth of those who need treatment receive it.

And what view did the government of the unlamented President Yanukovych take? On my first visit to Kiev, I interviewed the deputy health minister Oleksandr Tolstanov – the health minister herself becoming suddenly unavailable. As I continued in my questions about their policy on HIV, he turned to a colleague on his side of the table and asked in Russian (I had an interpreter): 'How much longer is this questioning going to continue?' He was more accustomed to the bland generalisations of an official visit. More significantly, when I asked about the lack of antiretroviral drugs he muttered, half under his breath, 'but I have cancer patients to look after'. In other words there is 'good disease' and 'bad disease', with HIV and Aids very firmly in the bad disease box.

Even if you leave human rights to one side, the trouble with this prejudice and disinterest is that Ukraine has one of the very worst HIV problems in Europe. It is inevitable. If you ignore the needs of high risk groups – men having sex with men, transgender people, injecting drug users, and sex workers – then the figures for infection are not going to do anything other than rise. The best estimate of the number living with HIV in Ukraine is probably about 300,000, with 25,000 new infections each year. The position is three or four times as bad as the position in Britain, although Britain has an appreciably bigger population. In the region, only Russia has a worse record. Many of those living with HIV are undiagnosed (around 100,000) and inevitably this means that there is the constant danger of the virus being spread further. It is the familiar story. If you are a gay man you will think twice and three times about volunteering when the results could easily leak out and lead to ostracism by neighbours and families and even the loss of a job.

Numerically, however, it is the injecting drug users who dominate the HIV figures. The best estimate is that there are about 300,000 injecting drug users, and many of these end up with HIV and even more with Hepatitis C. Officials explain that Ukraine is on the drugs route from Afghanistan – but that is not remotely the full explanation. The opium poppy is also grown in Ukraine itself and a lethal mixture of poppy extract and ingredients like baking soda and vinegar is injected. All told, there are around 125,000 criminal cases a year, with convictions involving the home-manufactured product far exceeding the pure heroin trade.

It all looks uncannily like the position in Russia. The same issues come up and the government all too often turns a blind eye to the gravity of the problem and spends all too little on containing the spread – although everyone from the Global Fund downwards tells them that they should spend more. But up to this point Ukraine has done what Russia increasingly refuses to do. It has allowed civil society organisations from other countries to help. The result is that a range of international organisations are at work here (like Alliance Ukraine and the Elton John Foundation) with the Global Fund providing much of the resource.

A small, overcrowded and cramped clinic by the side of the main road that goes north to Belarus provides an example of the gaping holes that these civil society organisations fill. The clinic provides what the government fails to – maintenance drugs to take users away from injecting. In the narrow corridor, a queue of drug users wait to see one of the nurses working here. In turn they take their place in a tiny, bleak room. The nurse dispenses not methadone but a tablet of an opioid called buprenorphine, which she has already crushed. She puts the powder into a thick piece of white paper shaped into a funnel and feeds it underneath the tongue of the patient. There is then a fifteen-minute wait which, among other things, is to prevent the drug being held in the mouth and sold outside. Tomorrow the patient will wait again in the corridor for his daily maintenance.

Some have been coming back for six or seven years – even longer – and the obvious question arises as to what, exactly, this treatment achieves. Dr Igor Antonenkov, the senior doctor at the clinic, points to the queue lining the corridor. 'There you see people who are not alcoholic, not injecting drugs, and not committing crime. They are relating better with their families and they are alive.' He adds that a third also have jobs. If they were back on the streets they would need to raise around a hundred dollars a day to continue their injecting habit from crime, together with all the dangers that go with it.

There is an even deeper justification for this method of treatment. 'The problem of using drugs is a disease of personality,' Dr Antonenkov says. 'The biggest problem is psychological dependence.' The aim is first to take them away from drugs on the street and then – if the will is there – to take them off drugs altogether. There is no predetermined timetable but, as well as two doctors and five nurses, there are two social workers and a psychiatrist at the clinic to help. At the clinic there was a woman who was now drug-free although her husband (who held down a good job) still needed the crutch of the daily visits. No one here would regard that as failure. It is an infinite advance on the blunt Russian methods, and on the crude ambitions of some politicians (rarely clinicians) further along the road to the West who still hanker for sudden cures.

The other major contribution that civil society organisations can make is value for money in a country where corruption still rules. Back in 2004 the Global Fund, in a highly unusual step, stopped its grant to the health ministry in Kiev on the suspicion that many of the funds were being siphoned off. The suspicions proved to be utterly well founded. Alliance Ukraine, part of the International HIV Alliance, took over the Global Fund contract. In one antiretroviral drug purchase they achieved an almost incredible reduction in price of twenty seven times – yes, *twenty-seven times*. How many lives were lost through this particularly nasty piece of corruption which had directly preyed on the ill?

It would be good to report that the corruption has now been eradicated from the medical system in Ukraine but so far that is not remotely the case. In 2013 a Ukrainian civil society organisation called the Anti-Corruption Action Centre monitored the public procurement of medicines for HIV and Aids and TB during the year. Their report was damning. It found that the government used 'limited existing resources to purchase medications at prices above market value. As a result thousands of critically ill Ukrainians do not receive the necessary therapy they need to survive. They have become hostages of a corrupt state procurement system.'

Among the abuses the centre found was that the tender process was strictly limited so that a $30 million budget was divided between six of the 6,500 pharmaceutical companies authorised for trading. There were false tenders that on the surface appeared to be between a number of companies but in fact were all controlled by one owner. Where there were different beneficiaries cartel arrangements could result in collusion between them. The bureaucracy left over from the Soviet period can also slow down or even halt the flow of medicines. In one recent case (separate from the centre's report) a consignment of syringes was held up at customs for several months. The syringes had been donated free but nevertheless the customs authorities wanted $200,000 before they would allow entry.

Of course all this is deeply against the public's interest. In the West and in Africa the history of treatment for HIV has been punctuated by fights between the civil society organisations and the big pharmaceutical companies. The heads of American foundations, like Bill Gates and Bill Clinton, are not the kind of men who will be intimidated into paying more than a fair price. In Ukraine the challenge has been to allow the civil society organisations to achieve the best possible deals. An example of what can be achieved was shown by Alliance Ukraine in 2013 when they negotiated an agreement with one pharmaceutical company which reduced the cost of a 48-week course for Hepatitis C by over half. Well over a million people are infected with Hepatitis C in Ukraine and, according to Andriy Klepikov, the organisation's executive director, 'we have managed to overcome the key obstacle when it comes to treatment – the price'.

This is at one end of the financial scale. On a more everyday basis, under-the-counter payments to medical staff are commonplace. I was surprised when I was told how chronically underpaid doctors and nurses appeared to be. Doctors could expect $300 a month and nurses $200. It would be more accurate, however, to say that for many this is their basic pay. It does not take into account the untaxed payments that are expected and required from patients at every turn. A patient entering a public hospital for an operation might well find that he is required to pay out between $300 and $400 to the staff. It is definitely not treatment that is free at the point of delivery. The doctors and nurses who *do* receive just their basic pay are the good people working in the modest clinic for drug users by the side of the road going north to Belarus.

To add to the difficulties another question beckons. At present the lion's share of the resources going to fight HIV comes from outside the country – most of all from the Global Fund in Geneva. But the Global Fund is looking at their priorities. Not unreasonably they want to concentrate resources on the poorest nations. Ukraine does not fit into this category. In the jargon of aid this is known as a 'mid-income' country. In Kiev you wait in long traffic queues with Range Rovers and Mercedes. There are placards for Aston Martins and Jaguars at the side of the road. I even spied a Ferrari showroom. But it is deceptive. The true position, according to one diplomat, is that 'there are too many oligarchs and too few middle class'. Subsistence farming sustains the population outside the capital. Given the political turmoil, it would be a particularly bad moment for the Global Fund to change its policy.

At the end of 2013 the position was that new HIV infections were continuing to increase, corruption was continuing to prevent resources reaching their proper destination of sick patients and there was the prospect of a cut in the already inadequate budget devoted to the epidemic. You might think that it could hardly get worse – but at the start of 2014 it did just that. On 17 January, as a direct response to the demonstrators of Independence Square, President Yanukovich signed into law a series of repressive measures which in practice were a giant step towards copying the public order controls of Russia. In Parliament, a total of eleven new laws were passed by shows of hands so rapid that they could not be counted. From the point of view of combating HIV, the most ominous development was the new law concerning civil society organisations. Just as in Russia, the proposal was that organisations that receive funds from overseas would need to be registered as 'foreign agents'. A barrier was being put up to the very international funds that had sustained the whole fight against HIV.

As the New Year advanced there seemed little reason for hope of progress. This, after all, was the government that had already imprisoned the former Prime Minister Yulia Tymoshenko and left her languishing for month after month in gaol. This was the government that has done all too little to tackle the endemic corruption that scarred the nation. And this was the government that not only looked the other way on the human rights of gay people but was quite happy to see their position exploited. Then in February 2014 the whole picture changed. The President was forced out of office after bloody battles in and around Independence Square. New elections were called. As I write, the final position remains uncertain.

In one respect, however, a division has already been drawn. One of the first actions of the Russian authorities in Crimea was to ban harm-reduction programmes and the use of opioids like methadone. The result is that almost a thousand unfortunate drug users have been thrown back on the tender mercies of the ineffectual Russian system. In Kiev, the harm-reduction policies remain, to the public benefit – and hopefully other beneficial policies can be developed.

New elections and a new government bring the opportunity of a new start. Any government in Ukraine will be told that their first tasks are to sort out the economy and corruption. But the tests are not just economic. Even in the years since independence in 1992 human rights have too often been trampled in the dust and prejudice has been allowed free rein. The opportunity now is for a fresh start that recognises the rights of gays and lesbians and other minorities to live free of official and public prejudice. If that could be achieved then the gain in tackling HIV and Aids would be immense. All governments should remember that the real test of a democracy is how you treat your minorities.

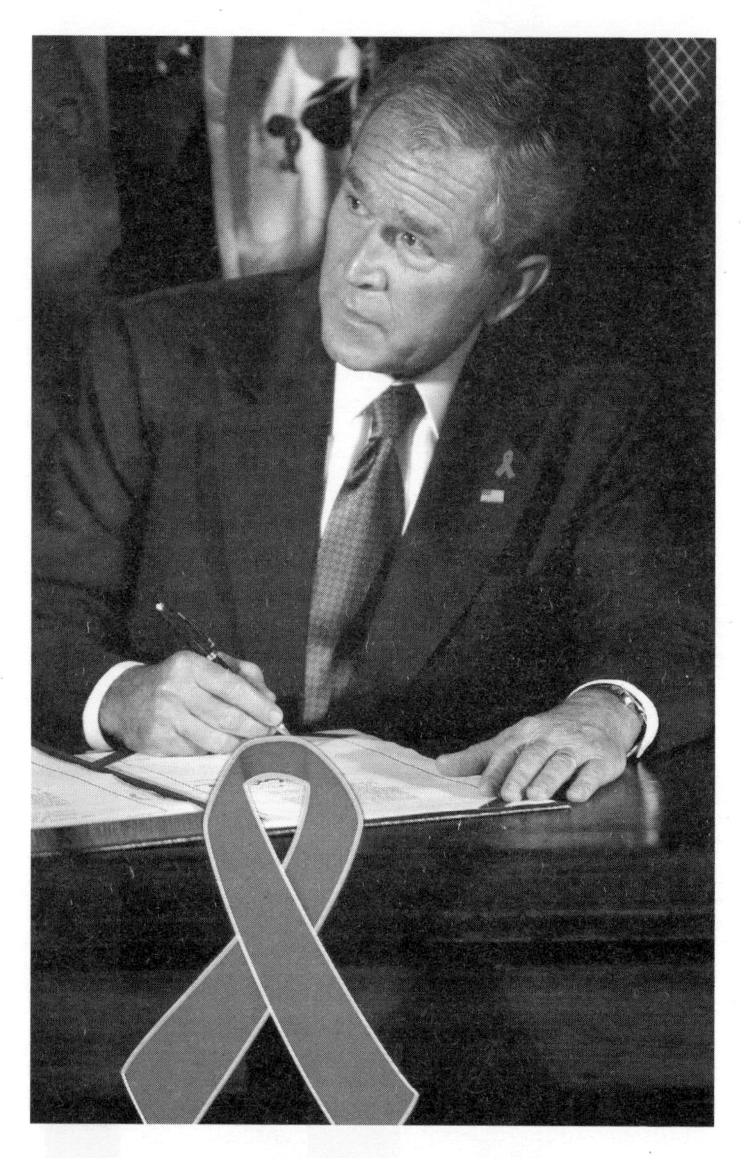

George Bush – the unlikely hero who was instrumental in providing help to combat Aids around the world.

SEVEN

WASHINGTON: A SHORT STEP FROM THE WHITE HOUSE

NO ONE CAN accuse the small organisation that has set up shop in Washington DC near to the Anacostia River and a couple of miles from the White House of being unclear about its objectives. With total frankness they proclaim their name – Help Individual Prostitutes Survive – and for the last twenty years that is exactly what they have done. They are there to help sex workers live a life free of infection, intimidation and violence. Their cavernous office is down a steep stairway in the basement of an unprepossessing office building next to a liquor store. A notice inside warns: 'Caution. Rat Traps Active Throughout'. They fight for funds to survive but this mixture of ex-sex workers – men, women and transgender – together with about fifty active volunteers run a service that, in one respect at least, does more for the public good than is achieved by quite a number of congressmen in their comfortable offices on Capitol Hill.

HIPS, as everyone calls it, is one of the main sources of clean needles for injecting drug users in the city. When I visited in June 2013, they told me that in the last twelve months they had distributed around 200,000 clean needles, often from a van that trundles the streets of Districts Seven and Eight between 8.00 at night and 5.00 the next morning – their hours follow the working hours of their clients. In the same twelve months they provided around a million condoms.

The United States is a nation of contradictions. Internationally they have brought massive help to countries who otherwise would not have been able to cope. Their aid has saved the lives of millions of men, women and children who a few years ago would have certainly died, and has stemmed the flow of the Aids orphans and the babies born with HIV. The money that they still devote to research holds out the greatest hope for the future. Their policies, for all the warts, are immeasurably superior to those of their old Communist foes. Their generosity is in an entirely different league. These are noble achievements, but the great irony is that America itself suffers from some of the same deficiencies that they spend billions of dollars trying to put right in other lands. Their present health insurance system is simply not fit for the purpose of tackling a public health epidemic like HIV and Aids. Some of their policies put political populism in front of what is necessary. Their general failure to engage with sex workers means that an obvious method of transmission remains open.

Prostitution remains a criminal offence in Washington, as it does in most of the United States, and the exploitation and persecution of sex workers has often characterised relations between police and sex workers in American cities. A 2012 report by Human Rights Watch on the position in New York, Los Angeles, San Francisco and Washington revealed widespread abuse. Many sex workers, particularly members of the transgender community, said that they had been stopped and searched for condoms while walking home or even waiting for a bus. As in Russia, possession of condoms was treated as an admission of guilt and the public health interest of reducing infection was utterly ignored. That is why a recent agreement between HIPS and the police in Washington DC that possession of a condom by itself would not be regarded as proof of prostitution is seen as such a step forward.

Cyndee Clay, the vivacious executive director of HIPS, has worked in Anacostia for the last seventeen years. She told me, 'We want sex workers to be safe, healthy and free of coercion and violence. The policy of criminalising sex work and drug-taking exacerbates the problem not reduces it. Across the board sex workers face discrimination and a lot of violence.' The criminal law, she added, does not help: 'You can get five months in gaol for a five-dollar sex act.' Their basement office is a place of refuge and advice without the formality and deterrence of official form-filling.

> *Ninety per cent of my clients do not want to be doing sex work. They have no other choice. But that doesn't mean you can't make their position better. You won't do that by simply saying our only object is to get you out of sex work. It's not realistic. If you want to give up then we will help you. If you don't we will also help you. We recognise the need to survive.*

What makes the success of HIPS remarkable is that much of their work appears to directly contradict the position of Congress itself. Take drugs as an example. In 1988, just as Britain and a number of other countries were introducing clean needles, the United States decided to go in an entirely different direction. No federal funds would be made available for needle and syringe schemes – overseas or at home. The usual argument was put forward that it would only condone and encourage crime. And then, in 2009, as the ban became more and more indefensible and when the Democrats took control of both the Senate and the House of Representatives, policy changed. Federal funds became available, much to the delight of activists and the satisfaction of the Obama administration. But almost before the ink had dried on the new agreement, the ban was restored.

The elections of 2010 (confirmed in 2012) saw the Republicans take control of the House of Representatives – and a new breed of Republicans at that. The traditional and pragmatic old guard gave way to a new Tea Party intake, some of whom opposed virtually any spending of taxpayer funds. Money for an organisation called Help Individual Prostitutes Survive, one which dealt with both drug taking and sex work, was definitely not on their agenda. In this kind of political climate there was no way that the funding of schemes to enable drug users to contain, but continue, their habit would survive. In the negotiations to get through the budget of 2011, funds for clean-needle schemes perished and the ban was restored. One Democrat insider (with unusual party political honesty) explained the position to me.

> *Very few Republicans supported the policy but neither did quite a number of Democrats. They simply disregarded the evidence that it doesn't increase drug use. 'Clean needles for drug addicts' doesn't resonate locally with the voters. Most people see it as an issue of crime. They believe that it will just encourage it.*

He could, of course, have been describing the official view in Moscow.

The change was watched with dismay by many public health campaigners. Insults flew. The mildest was that Congress with a Democratic Senate and a Republican House of Representatives was 'dysfunctional' and was peopled by congressmen who were 'off the wall'. Since the almost catastrophic breakdown of the talks with President Obama in the autumn of 2013 over the budget, such criticism, of course, has become commonplace.

The saving grace is that the United States has a federal system and, in spite of all the stones thrown at it, a flourishing democracy. States can – and do – do their own thing. 'You can't just press a switch and everyone will fall into line', one federal health official told me. States like California and New York, and over two dozen others, finance their own needle schemes or at least allow them to be privately financed. They are not going to take orders from Washington, particularly when all the evidence points the other way. 'If you don't have policies that target drug users and sex workers are you really serious?' one campaigner I spoke to demanded to know. Of course the other side of the coin is that states that do not support needle schemes – notably states in the south like Texas and Tennessee – can never be forced to run them.

The kind of mess you can get into by going the opposite route is amply illustrated over the border in Canada, where there is conflict between the provincial government in Vancouver and the national government in Ottawa. In the early 1990s Vancouver saw an explosive increase in drug use and by 1996 almost a third of injecting drug users were infected with HIV and 90 per cent with Hepatitis C. This was swiftly followed by what Dr Julio Montaner, the director of the British Columbia HIV Centre, calls 'an epidemic in overdose deaths'. One part of Vancouver's response was to set up a needle exchange scheme on a supervised site where users could bring in their own drugs and inject them in a safe environment. The scheme succeeded to such an extent that the local police brought drug users to the site and overdosing was virtually eliminated. It was not enough, however, to persuade the federal government, which objected – again on the grounds that it was condoning illegality – and then pursued Dr Montaner and his colleagues in the courts, to the extent of taking the battle to the Supreme Court. The government case was unanimously rejected in September 2011, but no one thinks that even now Ottawa has given up the battle.

In the shadow of the White House, Washington DC has been spared Vancouver's kind of power struggle and not even the new generation of Republicans look set to seek one. Washington is in fact a constitutional anomaly: it is not a state, and locals sometimes complain vociferously that they live in a kind of limbo under the control of Congress itself. Vehicle licence plates proclaim 'no taxation without representation' and residents lament that as they have no congressmen of their own (only a delegate) they are run by 'senators from Kansas'. To be fair, and luckily for HIPS, when it comes to clean needles, local decision-making prevails. Policy is the responsibility of the city council and the mayor. They set out the policy and approve the funds to be devoted to it. Of course this does not do away with the argument that the federal ban itself is utterly regressive and puts political gut feeling ahead of evidence and the overwhelming view of the American medical and public health professions. Domestically the practical effect has been to deprive dozens of schemes of much needed resources, leaving them with no other option but to try to raise the money locally.

Shortly after the ban was reinstated, the 2012 International Aids Conference was held in Washington DC and there the Secretary of State, Hillary Clinton, declared her ambition for the future of HIV/Aids prevention. The International Aids Conference is a unique occasion that brings together directors of foundations, workers on the ground in different countries, and government ministers from around the globe (although for some reason in 2012 British ministers decided to miss out on the most important conference in the HIV calendar – a discussion for a later chapter). In putting together the conference, one barrier had already been torn down. Many of the men and women who attended were living with HIV themselves and for over twenty years US policy had been to prevent such people from coming into the country. At long last the restriction was lifted. The delegates were rewarded with an array of star speakers from Elton John to Bill Gates but, in policy terms, the most important speaker by a mile was the Secretary of State herself. But she did not mention the change of policy. At the very least a word or two of explanation might have been expected. But there was nothing. Not a word. It was the elephant inside the conference hall.

Instead, Mrs Clinton's message was deliberately up-beat, designed to inspire the 20,000 delegates who had streamed into the vast convention centre and to catch the attention of the world's media. She told us she looked forward to the historic goal of 'creating an Aids-free generation': a generation in which virtually no child anywhere will be born with HIV; in which adults will be 'at significantly lower risk' of becoming infected, irrespective of where they lived; a generation in which 'if someone does acquire HIV' they will have access to treatment to prevent them developing Aids and passing on the virus. If you looked at the small print it was something less than a pledge to eliminate HIV and Aids, but it was a barn-storming performance all the same and one which brought the audience to its feet.

So just how near are we to attaining Mrs Clinton's declared goal of an Aids-free generation? Let us test that rhetoric, not in some far off country, but in Mrs Clinton's own Washington backyard in the District of Columbia. On the face of it the Washington position does not look so bad. There are certainly parts of the United States which appear to have far bigger problems. In New York, 130,000 live with HIV and in California and Florida the figures are just above and just below the 100,000 mark. The comparable figure for Washington DC is a mere 15,000. But then Washington is a tightly confined city with a total population of only 600,000. Once population size is compared with infections, the true position is revealed. The adult HIV prevalence rate of just under 3 per cent puts the capital of the richest country in the world on a par with sub-Saharan countries like Nigeria and Rwanda. It's fair to say that comparison is overdone to the extent that it is hardly sensible to compare prevalence in one relatively small city with whole countries, where the peaks of urban areas tend to be evened out by the troughs of the suburbs and the countryside. Nevertheless, no one would deny that over the years the city has faced a major public health crisis. As Mrs Clinton herself says, 'Washington today has the worst problem of any comparable city in the United States.'

There has never been any secret about where the epidemic is concentrated. It is not in the smart streets of Georgetown but in Districts Seven and Eight where HIPS is centred. It is an area which is literally off the tourist map and, in spirit if not geographical distance, a thousand miles from the tourist buses and the bookshops and cafés around Dupont Circle. Poverty is endemic, unemployment runs at almost 20 per cent and housing is poor and overcrowded. I remember years ago a Washington journalist referring to it deprecatingly as the 'Gold Coast' to mark out the high number of African Americans living there.

A more sympathetic portrait was painted by the journalist Ewen MacAskill in *The Guardian*. In July 2011 he wrote:

> *It is a world where some homes are in permanent darkness at night because electricity bills cannot be paid, where fathers take little or no responsibility for their children, where single mothers agonise over how they are going to find the money for school uniform, where drug dealers rule the night and the murder rate is high.*

Throughout the 1990s and the first years of the twenty-first century, the HIV position in Washington steadily deteriorated and the mayor and the council did all too little to combat the rise. It was not until 2005 that the full scandal was properly revealed. An independent watchdog organisation, the DC Appleseed Center for Law and Justice, reported that the annual rate of new Aids cases in Washington was believed to be ten times the national average. One estimate was that one out of every twenty residents was infected. The report charged that frequent changes in HIV leadership in the council's health department prevented consistent policy making, that testing and condom distribution were utterly insufficient, that both prevention and needle exchange programmes were dangerously weak and that the surveillance system providing information for the policy makers was not fit for purpose.

The Appleseed report was entirely damning but had one beneficial effect: the then mayor, Tony Williams, declared HIV to be his 'number one priority'. The uphill struggle to recovery slowly began. The Aids section of the health department was put under the direction of determined reformer Marsha Martin after a whole series of her predecessors came and went. When she took over in September 2005 there was no real data on the size of the epidemic and no proper figures had *ever* been collected about new infections. When I spoke with her in July 2013 she told me her guiding principle had been that 'if we communicated to the public that this was a serious problem then the public would respond'. And so it proved.

The new management launched a city-wide testing campaign: 'Come together DC – Get screened for HIV'. By 2008 the District was providing 73,000 tests – an increase of 70 per cent on the year before. Better surveillance revealed a population where over half of new infections occurred in gay and bisexual men, with African American men and women most highly affected. What also became clear was that (as in so many countries) about a fifth of those with HIV were undiagnosed, did not know their condition and, other things being equal, would continue to spread the disease.

The latest figures show that the figure for public-supported HIV tests has now climbed to around 125,000 a year. Tests are made available in pharmacies and even when renewing a driver's licence. As drivers wait to take their eye tests they are offered the HIV check as a matter of routine. This success has been achieved in spite of the predictable reluctance of some private general practitioners, in a dispute over fees, to carry out this essentially simple task – which in any event could be done at home. At the same time as increased testing, the American capital also experienced 'the rubber revolution', with the District distributing an ever-increasing number of condoms – male and female. Around 115,000 were given away in 2006, 1.5 million in 2008 and today the District distributes over 4.5 million a year.

The result is that, in the latest of their periodic reports, DC Appleseed holds up Washington as an example of what can be achieved. HIV surveillance has now become 'a national model', testing and condom distribution are both rated today as A minus, while a straight A goes to prison work where tests are offered to all inmates as they enter with only a 10 per cent refusal rate – offering a guide to the British prison authorities who are now belatedly following suit. So it would be good to report that the position on the ground in Washington has been transformed. And yet in one respect the position seems hardly to have moved at all. The prevalence of HIV in DC is marginally up on the position back in 2005 and is the rate which has led to all the African comparisons. But that figure comes with a massive health warning. The prevalence rate (the number living with HIV compared to population) is valuable for showing the number of people who need treatment, but in substantial part it is a retrospective picture.

The much more worrying position is the trend in new infections – the incidence rate – and the number of deaths from Aids. In 2012 in Washington there were over 800 people newly diagnosed – down on the 1,300 peak of a few years ago but stubbornly stuck at this level. The equivalent national figures for the whole of the United States show some 50,000 people newly diagnosed each year – similarly stuck after the initial fall. As for deaths, the latest figures show that in Washington there are now around 200 deaths a year from Aids while nationally the figure is 15,500 a year – bringing the number of people who have died from Aids since the epidemic began to almost 650,000. Some find that a surprise: a few weeks before my visit to Washington in 2013 I was at Westminster, and was asked by a well-known and bright peer: 'Do people in the West still die from Aids?' He knew they died in Africa but could not conceive that it could still be the case in a rich country like the United States with all the modern drugs at their disposal.

For all the success that testing programmes have had in Washington it remains the case that thousands of men and women will still not come forward, with the result that much HIV remains undiagnosed. The stigma around HIV remains strong – particularly in the African American community. As Greg Pappas, who acquired a wealth of experience in his time at the District of Columbia health department told me, 'People die rather than face up to the fact that they are HIV positive.' Others simply do not want to reveal that they are gay and fear that the news could reach their family or neighbourhood. So to persuade more to test remains a difficult challenge – but there is another issue which raises just as many problems.

The comforting assumption is that if only you can get people to test then all problems are solved. It is assumed that if found positive they will automatically go onto treatment and just as automatically they will follow the regime and ensure a stable life. Sadly that is not remotely the case. Public health officials in Washington love to illustrate the issue with a 'cascade' chart which shows not only the difficulties of getting people into treatment but, once there, retaining them. The goal is full adherence to the treatment schedule and the achievement of minimal activity of the virus. This is termed an 'undetectable viral load' – which in plain English means more or less total suppression of the virus for the individual, which reduces infectiousness and the risks of HIV being passed on to other people.

That is the goal, but the official health figures tell a very different story. Out of almost 1.2 million people in the United States living with HIV, the figures cascade downwards to show little more than a quarter of that number with an undetectable viral load. A fifth are undiagnosed and live in ignorance of their condition. The cascade continues downwards with about 420,000 on antiretroviral treatment and, in the end, only 330,000 fully adhere to the treatment and have an undetectable viral load. The cascade is illustrated in the chart below:

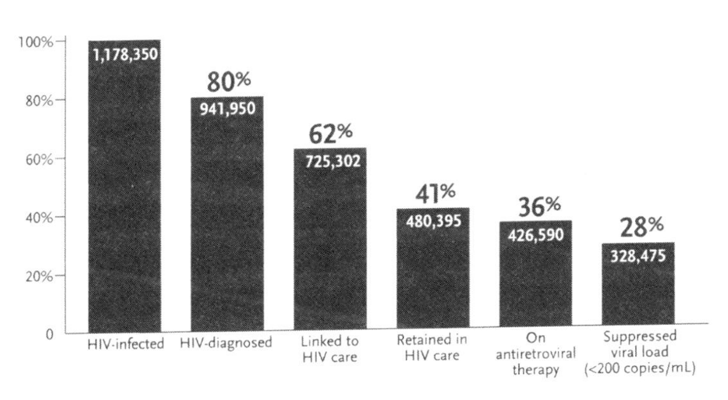

Source: CDC

In Washington the figures show the same trend. The figures of course are an average and in San Francisco, for example, the claim is that the drop-out rate is much less among men who have sex with men. But their achievement entails twenty-five years of fairly relentless publicity and (perhaps above all) an acceptance of gay sex which is not shared in much of the United States, let alone in very many other countries around the world.

The more general truth is that ensuring that patients adhere to the treatment is often every bit as difficult as persuading them into testing and treatment in the first place. Yet unless that is achieved a whole fresh set of complications arise. People risk death if they abandon treatment altogether, but more commonly they dip in and dip out. The problem for them is that they risk becoming drug resistant to the basic antiretroviral drugs and need more complex treatment which may or may not be available. The problem for the public is that the people who have dropped out of treatment become infectious again and can then spread the virus.

The American position pinpoints a major under-reported global issue. It shows what happens if access and adherence to treatment breaks down. If this happens in the richest of rich countries, what happens in the poorer countries of the world where health systems are under-developed and where there can be substantial difficulty for the patient in making the journey to the hospital in the first place? In the United States, apart from some remote areas, there are no physical obstacles in reaching medical care. Rather, the obstacles appear to be principally financial. Health care in the United States relies on private insurance but that leaves substantial numbers of uninsured or partially insured people who drop out of HIV care because they cannot afford to continue. This, after all, is why President Obama has expended so much political capital trying to reform health care with the Affordable Care Act. Men and women with HIV figure prominently among the uninsured and are potential beneficiaries. Or at least that is the hope. The latest study conducted at the beginning of 2014 by the Kaiser Family Foundation shows that the new act is unlikely to transform the position on HIV and Aids. Around 70,000 people with HIV *could* gain new coverage but that number will be reduced when the many states that do not plan to expand their Medicaid programmes are taken into account.

In contrast (as the table below shows) almost 60 per cent of those living with HIV across the Atlantic in Britain stick with their treatment and do not drop out. Britain runs the much maligned free-at-the-point-of-use National Health Service, which is attacked in the United States as a peculiarly socialist measure and sniped at in Britain for its well-reported failures. The central principle of the British health service is that no one is turned away from treatment for lack of funds. In public health, all logic tells you that should be the guiding principle. In the same way, France runs a much-admired health system which again produces a much wider coverage of antiretroviral therapy than anything reached in the United States. I should add a rider. The European figures are undoubtedly better, but they still show that 40 per cent of those with HIV (including the undiagnosed) have not achieved the goal of an undetectable viral load.

	Number with HIV	*% diagnosed*	*Retained in HIV care*	*On ART*	*Undetectable viral load*
UK	94,900	77%	73%	64%	58%
France	150,200	81%	74%	64%	56%
USA	1.17 million	80%	41%	36%	28%

So where does all this leave the United States in achieving Mrs Clinton's Aids-free generation? Some considerable way off I fear. Of course it is the case that the most massive progress has been made. We are light years from the position I saw in 1987 when young men were dying and the politicians were looking the other way. The position was turned around by men like the former surgeon general Everett Koop who came to Washington with a reputation as an unyielding moral conservative much loved by President Reagan and the White House and left as one of the most effective Aids campaigners the United States has ever known, much to the delight of the liberals who had vociferously opposed his appointment. In Washington DC enormous credit goes to Marsha Martin who, by reorganising the city's public health response, did so much to stem the tide in the capital itself and who now seeks to assist other cities in taking charge of their own epidemics. In addition there is an array of private foundations and civil society organisations which have been giving help ever since Washington's dark days; organisations like N Street Village and Whitman-Walker Health, which I will come to shortly, and of course HIPS. As Marsha Martin herself told me, 'If we did not have the private sector response it would be a nightmare. You cannot rely on government to provide the resources.'

Nevertheless the problems of reaching the Aids-free goal are formidable. Habits are slow to change and the impact of health promotion can wear off as the years go by. Most high-school-aged young people and a large number of children in middle school are sexually active. In Washington, over 13 per cent report having had sexual intercourse before the age of thirteen – over double the national average – and many have a number of partners. The use of condoms drops from 79 per cent for 14–17-year-olds to 45 per cent for 18–24-year-olds and the trend continues into middle age with inevitable results. In the US generally most new infections are among men and women in their twenties (15,500 per year) but they remain high with people in their thirties (11,500) and their forties (11,300) – those who have lived through at least a decade of prevention publicity. The US national figures show that of those people diagnosed 30,573 were infected from male to male sexual contact, about 3,600 from injecting drugs and 13,300 through heterosexual contacts – and in Washington the proportion of infections through heterosexual sex is higher than the national average. As one worker told me, 'The woman may be in a monogamous relationship but that does not mean the partner is doing the same.'

And there is one further overarching problem – deprivation. The head of one civil society organisation told me, 'The greatest barrier to preventing HIV is poverty. The next greatest is not to have medical insurance.' A local health official added 'We are not dealing with the educated middle class. We are dealing with people with a whole range of other issues like unemployment and homelessness.' Only a handful of those entitled to housing assistance in Washington receive it. According to a *Washington Post* report in April 2013, the average public housing wait for a one-bedroom apartment was twenty-eight years. Homelessness has been long associated with increased risky behaviour and poor health, while housing instability means simply communicating with people moving from one poor address to another is difficult and is an obvious barrier to both testing and treatment.

One significant effort to make progress is made by a private charity called N Street Village which cares for homeless women. Their origins go back almost twenty years to a time when they were the first to give care to homeless women in Washington who were dying from Aids. The director Schroeder Stribling told me, 'They faced terrible prejudice. Other women in a homeless hostel would say, "We don't want you here. We don't want to eat with you. We don't want to share your laundry." We said to the women: "You can stay here. You can die here."' Since then, with the new drugs, the position has changed radically, and inside the buildings of N Street Village much wider care is now provided. 'We didn't need full time nurses any more', she continued.

> *We needed to provide health and welfare services and to tackle addiction and mental illness. We are not so much dealing with women with kids but with women of forty and fifty. They have often suffered violence and are trying to find a safe place. They are exhausted. Their self-esteem is low and they suffer from depression. They need social support.*

The effects of homelessness and poverty in Washington go wide. Young gay black men face the prospect of being thrown out of their family home if their sexual orientation is revealed. They then need a roof over their head and it is at that point that they can get together with an older man and become infected. According to Don Blanchon, the head of Whitman-Walker Health, housed in the Elizabeth Taylor Medical Center (so called not because she started it, but because the original benefactor admired her as an actor), they do not have the power to insist on the use of a condom. In spite of all the efforts, the goal of a sensible standard of living and individual and family stability in Washington is still a long way off in Districts Seven and Eight. As Schroeder Stribling remarked, 'We are the nation's capital. We have all this power, all this money. And even then we don't get it done.' To put the point in the terms of this book: if it cannot be achieved in the capital of the richest nation on earth what chance is there in a slum in India, a township in South Africa, or a grindingly poor village in Ukraine? The answer is that the chances would be even less without American help.

For Washington does have another vastly important role. It is the political home for the biggest givers of international aid in the world. Washington funds the President's Emergency Plan for Aids Relief, known everywhere as PEPFAR, and USAID, which implements much of the work overseas. In the five years from 2009 to 2013 Congress authorised $48 billion of US taxpayers' money for the President's fund and, in addition, each year (and here they have to date proved entirely constructive) provide about a third of the revenue which enables the Global Fund to Fight Aids, Tuberculosis and Malaria to function. In both Washington and New York there is again an array of civil society organisations ranging from the International Aids Vaccine Initiative to the private foundations of Bill and Melinda Gates and of George Soros. But it is PEPFAR that is the most striking achievement. Countering HIV has never been the most popular cause among politicians and yet since 2003 the United States has sustained a vastly expensive programme giving help to people who, if the truth is known, are strongly disapproved of by many of the citizens of middle America. What is more it was a programme introduced by a Republican President.

PEPFAR was not the brain child of Hillary Clinton's husband when he was the United States President at the end of the 1990s. Bill Clinton did relatively little in the international field when he was actually in the White House. His daughter Chelsea is said to have asked him after he had left, 'Why didn't you do anything about global HIV?' Whether this is true or not, what is certain is that Bill Clinton's major contribution came – like President Mandela in South Africa – after he had left office, with the Clinton Foundation and his formidable success in bringing down the price of drugs. Nevertheless, the author of the emergency fund which has saved countless lives was his Republican successor George W. Bush. Much reviled for the 'War on Terror' and the invasion of Iraq, it is probably his greatest legacy. As Jason Wright, the head of International HIV/Aids Alliance in Washington, told me, 'It was a sort of Nixon goes to China thing. It was crucial that it was a Republican President doing this. The Republicans supported their President.'

The figures spelling out the achievements since then are by any standards impressive. The United States, through PEPFAR, now supports over six million people around the world on antiretroviral treatment – up from 1.7 million in 2008 – and each year provides drugs to prevent mother-to-child transmission for around 1.5 million pregnant women. The goal is to reach a position where the numbers put onto treatment in individual nations each year at least exceed the new HIV infections. That process has still a long way to go. In countries like Botswana and Kenya treatment is ahead of new infections but in others, like Nigeria and Uganda, it is vastly behind.

Some critics say that although the US spends a vast amount on countering Aids, its total spend on overseas aid is still only 0.2 per cent of GDP, compared with the 0.7 per cent which is the United Nations' goal and which countries like Britain make a particular effort to meet. But as a former British Chancellor of the Exchequer, Nigel Lawson, was apt to say, 'cash is cash' and for the last fifteen years American cash has kept poor nations supported and international organisations financed. A more fundamental criticism is that some of the conditions laid down over the years for the receipt of funds have been unnecessarily and damagingly restrictive.

One rule laid down is that PEPFAR must report to Congress if a country fails to spend sufficient of its prevention funding to 'promote abstinence, delay of sexual debut, monogamy, fidelity and partner reduction'. Reports still faithfully record the number of abstinence messages that are distributed. When I was in Kenya just after the New Year in 2013, I was handed a report that said around 720,000 people were reached with 'abstinence and faithfulness messages' in 2011. The suspicion is that, although sincere, these efforts are no more successful than the efforts of the British and Canadian armies in the First World War that exhorted soldiers to 'do your duty, fear God and honour the King'. As many workers point out, abstinence for women is little use if the men they eventually team up with are HIV positive. Nevertheless the 'no grazing', 'keep to one partner' messages which aim to break the habit of multiple partners can be useful – provided they are seen to come from national politicians and health officials rather than from overseas.

An undoubtedly damaging PEPFAR rule concerns sex workers. Historically grants have always come with two conditions. First funds cannot be used to 'promote or advocate' the legalisation of prostitution and second grants can only go to groups with a policy which 'explicitly' opposes prostitution. There has then been a policy requirement that organisations tackling HIV must refrain from any speech or activity that the government deems 'inconsistent' with the anti-prostitution pledge. That has extended to what a recipient says or does not only with PEPFAR funds but even with its own private funds.

Not surprisingly these rules have put successive administrations under fire from civil society organisations and, at last, in June 2013 that flak led to a successful legal challenge. The Supreme Court ruled that the First Amendment to the Constitution precluded the government not only from censoring speech but also from 'telling people what they must say'. However, whether the Supreme Court decision has settled the issue is quite another matter. The ruling applies only to United States organisations and not to foreign-based ones, and there still remains the power of any government to choose to fund some activities and not others.

And so we return to the elephant in the room at the International Aids Conference in 2012. Perhaps the Secretary of State failed to mention the renewed ban on using federal funds for needle schemes because overseas, where alternative funding is not easy to come by, the impact of the government's backflip will be much more severe. With casualties from injecting drugs still rising in Eastern Europe and Central Asia and with drugs now making an unwelcome appearance in Africa, it is a decision that goes smack against all the good work that the United States has done internationally over the last years.

They gave Mrs Clinton a standing ovation that day because everyone in that vast Washington hall believed that in terms of HIV and Aids the United States had saved the world and that without their effort a whole range of countries would be in an utterly desperate plight today. They also wanted to believe that the historic goal of an Aids-free generation was near but – uneasily – they recalled the world as they knew it: the vast distance there was still to travel in Africa; the deteriorating position in Russia and Eastern Europe; the sheer numbers infected in India and China; the ominous signs of new epidemics in the Middle East and North Africa; and the depressing statistic that, even today, for every new person put on treatment many more are infected. Some thought that she was being optimistic, others that she was falsely raising expectations

– rather like the periodic newspaper headline promising 'a cure to Aids'.

The obstinate refusal of too many American politicians to help drug users means that dirty needles still spread the epidemic not only at home but in other countries of the world. None of this is the fault of the clinicians, the local health workers, or the volunteers. The fault lies fairly and squarely with the politicians. It is political action which is required: political action in Washington. If the politicians were to look again at just the ban on supporting clean-needle schemes that would help not only the American public but also send a clear message around the world. As it is, Russian officials now claim that the United States has been converted to their harsh and balefully unsuccessful policies. Can Republican congressmen (together with some Democrats) be happy that they are now portrayed in the world as arm in arm with Russian officials, following the old Communist ways? Are they content to bring up the rear in this particular conga of death?

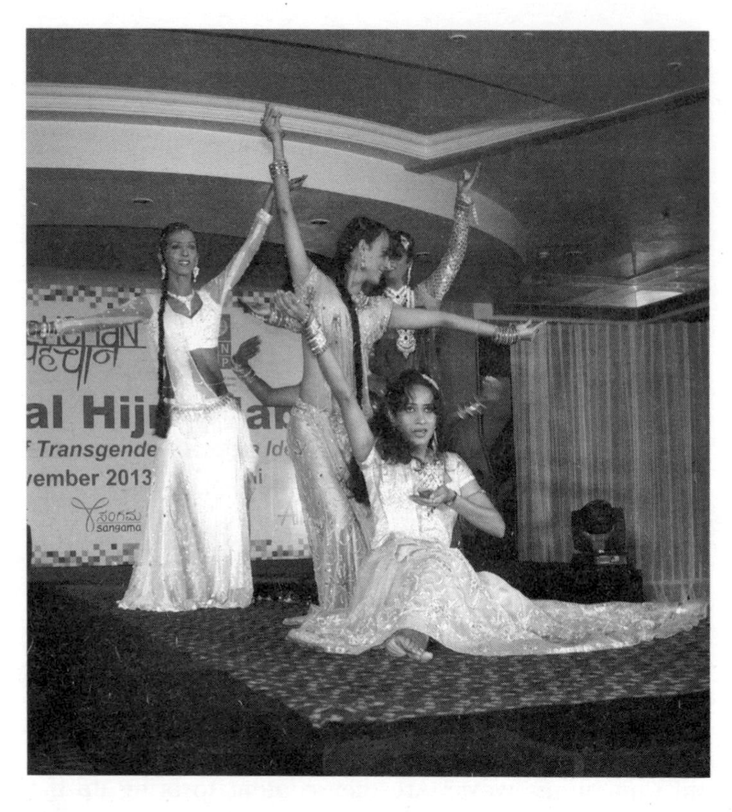

Hijra *dancers perform at a 2013 rally to support transgender people, one of the most marginalised groups in India.*

EIGHT

NEW DELHI: 1860 AND ALL THAT

THERE IS ONE group in India which probably suffers more discrimination than any other minority in this vast sub-continent. They are effectively barred from most jobs. It is not that they fail the interview – they are turned away at the gate. They face the equivalent of the 'no blacks' notices displayed by some landladies in Britain in the 1950s. On public transport, passengers move to another seat if one happens to sit next to them. They are very often rejected by their own families, subject to violence and are even lower down the notoriously caste-ridden Indian social scale than the 'untouchables'. They are the transgender people, and they are also the group with the highest rate of HIV.

With normal employment opportunities largely excluded, options for earning any sort of living are severely limited. Begging is one option, and this is not just a matter of holding out a begging bowl. The begging is much more organised than that. *Hijras* have a long recorded history on the Indian sub-continent and historically have been the face of the transgender population. In his portrait of Delhi, *City of Djinns*, William Dalrymple describes how, after weeks of gradual persuasion, he was allowed to go out early one morning with three *hijras* accompanied by two musicians. Dalrymple's group lived together in a small household under the guidance of an older *guru*, who directed them to a list of local weddings that she had put together. Although in the Hindu tradition *hijras* are viewed with disdain, they are also treated with caution and some superstition. In particular, newlyweds do not want a possible 'curse' hanging over them. The result is that the *hijras* dance as the musicians play and the guests and the neighbourhood watch. They withdraw only when the *guru* has extracted the desired amount of money from the family.

Another income opportunity for a transgender person is to work as a dancer in a bar. The last option is to become a sex worker. Many are forced to choose this last way. The younger you are the higher the price, and there are stories of young boys being castrated so that the family can take advantage of his earning power. This, however, is not remotely typical. For most, the journey is entered into voluntarily, in spite of all the difficulties and dangers. The practicalities are perilous. Few doctors will carry out a castration operation. The result is that they are at the mercy of the quack. Operations are done without proper hygiene and the fact that about one in ten die as a result tells its own story. Operations are not cheap. Castration would cost anywhere between 20,000 and 60,000 rupees. That is between about $330 and $1,000 when much of the Indian population live on a few dollars a day. Vaginal construction surgery could cost well over double that and there is also the added cost of hormonal treatment. So why do Indian transgender people spend the money and take the risk?

When I visited India in November 2013, I met Abhina Aher, now a good looking woman in her late thirties and invariably dressed in bright colours, who told me, 'Transgender women want to be beautiful women. Unless you are castrated then the others look down on you.' At one stage she worked with a gay organisation but said: 'I did not want to be loved as a man. I wanted to be loved as a woman with children.' The whole of this ambition may have eluded her but, like all the transgender people I met, she is happy as she is. She remembers clearly enough the struggles to get to where she is today.

As a young boy of about six or seven she became certain that she was in the wrong body. Her father had died when she was three and, without encouragement, she began to copy her mother who was a dancer. Looking back today she says she 'got a kick' from wearing her mother's clothes, her jewellery and her dancing equipment. On one occasion she was found by her mother dressed up in this way but was roundly told: 'You are a boy. Boys don't dance.'

According to Abhina, her overwhelming problem was a lack of understanding and a lack of information. Sex was taboo. 'You could not talk to anyone about it. You could not talk to your family. You could not talk to your teachers.' The one time she complained to her teachers about the treatment she was receiving from her classmates, she was told that it was she who was responsible because of the effeminate way she behaved. The only early medical advice she received (if such it can be called) was from a doctor in a public hospital, who said that she should 'sleep in a dark room' so that she could come to terms with herself.

In her late teens she made three attempts at suicide. 'It was a mixture of loneliness and rejection. I felt I had no role in the world. Self-pity took over.' For several years she took no action. She told me she was shocked at being approached by a *hijra* and asked for money. 'If I am like her I don't want to end up a beggar,' she said. Instead, she studied and was employed in a software programming company. It was only when, through a lonely hearts magazine, she found others who felt the same that she started on changing her life. She is now successfully employed, giving both men and women the support and information that she was denied. She says that her mother still does not understand, but nevertheless she supports her. 'We are linked by blood,' her mother told her. 'I am going to be with you. I gave you birth.' It is a happier family outcome than for many others.

Another transgender woman who has followed the same course is Simran Sheikh. She ran away from home when she was fourteen after suffering years of mockery inside her middle-class family. For three days she sat outside Mumbai railway station without food or water. 'Those three days were the toughest time of my life,' she told me. 'I didn't want to go back but I didn't know where to go.' Finally she was befriended by a *hijra* who took her home and, over the next months, taught her the basics of her new life. She worked for about five years dancing in bars, but that was brought to an end when the bars in Mumbai were forced to close in 2005. Sex work became the only option and she worked in the red-light area, Kamati Pura, but continued with her education and joined the first ever transgender organisation in 1999. Like Abhina she now works to help others and, also like Abhina, has no regrets about the change. As for her family, she tried once to ring them but was told, 'You are dead for us.'

It is, of course, this isolation that makes transgender people so vulnerable – and so vulnerable to HIV. At 8.8 per cent, their HIV prevalence is dramatically higher than that for the general public. One reason is that they are in a peculiarly weak position to insist on men using a condom. Unprotected sex is overwhelmingly the main route of transmission in India. Another reason is the discrimination against them in the medical system. Even doctors can make clear their distaste. 'Go over there,' they say. 'We will see you at the end.' This all adds up to giving transgender people an understandable reluctance to test and a reluctance to seek advice on other sexual diseases which could increase their vulnerability to HIV.

India shows the kind of response that transgender people (who also include the much smaller number who transition from female to male) receive around the world. To an outsider like me, the discrimination and heartache is difficult to understand. All the transgender community wants is to be recognised and treated just like anyone else. As Simran told me, 'We want to be accepted.' It is hardly an unreasonable request. It is the cry of every persecuted group over the ages. Transgender people may be the least known of the sexual minorities, but for some their very appearance seems to provoke revulsion – which is ironic given that they are often better turned out and better dressed than their orthodox counterparts.

On the last evening of my visit to Delhi, I went to an event which fell somewhere between a gay pride celebration and a political rally. A long catwalk protruded from the stage into the audience as the *hijra* dancers in their brightly coloured saris went skilfully through their complex routines in a blaze of purple, scarlet and yellow. Impeccable performances were punctuated by speeches calling for action. A government secretary promised reform, a well-known Bollywood film actor pledged support. The 300-strong audience responded with enthusiasm and the hope that India is seeing the beginning of a new age. That is the hope, but a thousand years of discrimination may not be ended that easily. The prospect is that, for the foreseeable future, many transgender people will continue to be forced into sex work – and their rate of HIV infection will continue to be high.

Of course, given the size of the Indian population, you could argue that the plight of the minority transgender population is something of a side show. Estimates of the number of transgender people vary enormously. The figures I heard ranged from 160,000 at the lowest to 750,000 at the highest. Certainly the National Aids Control Organisation in New Delhi argue their case on a larger canvas – and so would I if I had to cope with a population of 1.2 billion spread over twenty-eight different states and six union territories, as well as the region around Delhi itself. India is not a centralised country like China. You cannot issue instructions here and expect that they will be observed to the letter everywhere from Calcutta to Mumbai. Nevertheless India claims very substantial success in checking the spread of HIV.

There may be over two million people with HIV in India but, when population is taken into account, that means the prevalence is under 0.3 per cent. This is not only way below the figures in sub-Saharan Africa but also rich countries like the United States. If only South Africa or Nigeria could have achieved such results then the world epidemic would have been dramatically less. New infections are estimated to be down to 130,000 a year – a reduction of half over the last decade. Government figures also suggest that deaths from Aids have reduced to around 150,000 a year which is again a big improvement on the position ten years ago. There are some observers who think that the official figures are too sunny but nevertheless no one can doubt the progress that has been made.

As for treatment there again has been progress. About 600,000 patients living with HIV are receiving antiretroviral drugs but that still leaves a massive number either not on treatment or unaware that they have HIV in the first place. Some clinicians make no bones about the position and admit that many will die waiting. Then there is the added problem of adherence, with many finding the difficulty and expense of travelling to a hospital to be almost prohibitive. The result is that one estimate suggests that as many as a third do not stick with their treatment.

Prevention, however, is India's proudest boast. According to Aradhana Johri, Additional Secretary of National Aids Control Organisation, India is 'a global success' in preventing Aids. India, she told me, 'has focused on prevention'. The government has led from the front, and the result has been 'the world's largest mass mobilisation campaign'. So let us examine just how much of a global leader India is and how successful it has been. To what extent is this, the largest democracy in the world, an example to us all?

What sets India apart has been the general consistency of their policy, their emphasis on prevention and the fact that they acted early. They did not wait until they had been partly overwhelmed before responding. The National Aids Control Organisation was formed back in 1992 and is now just embarking on its fourth five-year plan. Even sceptics of national plans might concede their success. In that time, condoms have been promoted in a country which, despite the sexually explicit statues and erotic friezes that can be found, often does not talk openly of sex. A clean-needles policy was introduced early and public health was put firmly in front of the misguided fears that it would lead 'inevitably' to a rise in crime. Every opportunity has been taken in prevention publicity, including the Red Ribbon Express, a special train running through India taking condoms and the public health message to small towns and villages. At the same time, India has progressively taken over responsibility for financing both treatment and prevention from international donors.

By any standards these are impressive achievements, but there remain formidable problems to overcome. India says it has a 'concentrated epidemic', by which it means that the dangers are concentrated in the high risk groups – sex workers, injecting drug users, men who have sex with men and of course transgender people and *hijras*. There is no complete agreement on the numbers except that the figures are massive. One official survey in 2007 estimated that there were around three million female sex workers – and that leaves aside an unknown but potentially substantial number of male sex workers. Human Rights Watch put the number of sex workers substantially higher than anything in official reports, but everyone is agreed that women in particular who have embarked on this course find it next to impossible to change their lives.

Another survey estimated that there were over 2,300,000 men who regularly have sex with other men, but again this is thought to be a substantial under-estimate. In addition there are significant transient groups who can easily spread the virus. There are well over two million long-distance truckers moving throughout the country – away from their families and the restraints of their communities. Huge numbers of Indians also migrate within the country, leading unstable lives distant from the health system. They move to where the work is. The area around Surat in Gujurat is one such magnet, where the high employment opportunities in the local industries attract migrants from poorer states, who then live in makeshift shacks by the side of the road. Connecting with all these groups is a mammoth task.

And then of course there are injecting drug users. The overall number of drug users is unknown, although government figures suggest that there are almost 200,000 drug users who inject. In Delhi one survey showed that their HIV prevalence was over 20 per cent – over double the figure for injecting drug users nationally. Not only are they continuing to increase in numbers, the drugs they inject continue to change. Once, the problem centred on heroin and was concentrated in the north east of the country, near China and on the border with Myanmar (Burma that was). Today it is much more widespread and more complex. The biggest problem is the misuse of pharmaceutical products that can be bought over the chemist's counter. 'You can go into a pharmacy and can get more or less anything you want,' one outreach worker explained to me. A well-known antihistamine is a favourite ingredient in the mixture. Although everyone realises what is happening, the police do not intervene and the trade continues. The heavy suspicion is that money has changed hands. It is all too reminiscent of the home-made drugs position in Moscow, but different in one vital respect. India not only allows clean-needle policies, it also finances them. But this comes with a health warning: anyone who thinks that this implies sterilised conditions, spotlessly clean injecting rooms and nurses in white uniforms should think again.

By the side of the Yamuna-Bazar River on the outskirts of Delhi there is a treatment centre that, when I visited it in 2012, reminded me of something straight from the pages of Charles Dickens. The centre is on a large untidy site bounded on one side by the river. Emaciated men stand listlessly in small groups. A few yards away a young man in a filthy shirt and cap is injected by another user wearing an old track suit top. An old man is being treated for an abscess brought on by his injecting habit. A young boy of fourteen or fifteen, who I'm told started injecting himself a year previously, looks up from a rudimentary lesson a helper is giving him. As he is under eighteen he, like many others, will not appear in the official statistics. At night there is a spartan shelter for up to a hundred drug users, who are packed into the space, sleeping side by side on the bare floor with a ration of one blanket each. Drug users raise what funds they can from rag picking or, even better, from collecting empty cans, for which they can expect a price of between 50 and 200 rupees. Sacks full to the brim are stored at the corner of the site.

In the main building itself a small queue forms outside what might be called the dispensary. This sets out to help users who are trying to come off injecting altogether. A helper marks off each name and then, one by one, they are seen by the nurse who starts work each day at 8 a.m. and carries on into the early evening. The nurse grinds the tablets (buprenorphin) and feeds the powder to the users. As in Kiev, there is no question of simply handing over a full tablet – it might be taken away and sold. For the same reason the users are required to wait for fifteen minutes before leaving.

You wonder how a system like this can produce success, but it does. In 1998 HIV prevalence among the clinic's clients was 44 per cent. Today only 11 per cent of the current injecting drug users are infected. Much of this improvement is due to the utter dedication of the staff and the civil society organisations that carry out this work. Some of the staff are former drug users themselves. 'If you have not experienced this yourself then you don't know what they are feeling,' one of the workers on the site told me. Other staff, like the dispensary nurse who has worked on the site year after year, are just examples of pure dedication. To come in each day to what is little more than a kiosk and then to minister to an endless line of drug users – some of whom are on the look-out for an opportunity to smuggle out the drug – requires a dedication which few possess. It is just as well such people and such organisations exist for without them the figures would not look anything like as good.

Another priority group are the sex workers and here Indian officials take particular pride in the fact that the national prevalence has reduced to 2.4 per cent a year. Certainly that has nothing to do with the clarity of the law. The regulation of prostitution is the usual muddle to be found in most countries around the world. The exchange of sexual services for money is legal but (and it is a very big 'but') soliciting in a public place, owning or managing a brothel, pimping and kerb crawling are all criminal offences. In practice the uncertainty leaves the way open for exploitation, including exploitation by the police.

In a small house in a dingy part of West Delhi I interviewed a group of four sex workers. They were in their thirties or forties. All had children, and that was their priority. One woman told me, 'There was no choice. My husband left. You have to live somehow.' Sometimes they have been very successful. A small woman in a pink sari said that she had financed her son through Delhi University, although often as they grow up the children turn against their mothers and their way of life.

I asked, what was their main problem? Almost in unison they complained of their pimps. The pimp would probably be an ex-sex worker herself. She would rent a house and have a pool of between ten and fifteen women who lived locally who would come in most days. They would have ten clients during the day and for that the pimp would be paid about 2,000 rupees. Out of this sum the sex worker would receive 200. Condoms would usually be used but if the client wanted sex without it then the pimp would agree to what the client wanted. The sex worker would be in no position to refuse.

Not all sex work in this part of Delhi was organised this way. Others worked in the local Chameli Park. 'The younger you are, the better,' said one of the women I interviewed. A fourteen- or fifteen-year-old (possibly the daughter of a sex worker herself) might be paid up to 1,000 rupees for a day's work. Like the young drug users, at under eighteen she also would not appear in the official statistics. There was one other point on which the women were united. They would never go to the police for help. 'I have never even tried,' said one. The police are viewed as both corrupt and violent. The sex workers' plea was: 'Tell the police not to exploit us. They come every week asking for money. They keep coming back.' It is the all too common global problem.

The position here cries out for reform. By common consent, the whole system is shot through with corruption and the violence of gangsters, who demand protection money, or of clients who for one reason or another are dissatisfied and refuse to pay. You would think that any logical policy would demand some form of proper control which would not only be good for the sex workers but also benefit the cause of public health. But this would also mean official regulation of sex work and, like so many other countries around the world, India has no intention of travelling down that path. The politicians would not accept such a solution – and neither would the religious leaders.

The vast majority of the country is Hindu (about 80 per cent) and after that come Muslims (about 13 per cent). If you were to generalise (which is a perilous venture in this vast nation) you would say that India is a religiously conservative country where most of the population engage in religious rituals on a daily basis. Religious conflicts periodically break out: the worst by far being the widespread riots and murders in the years around Indian independence in 1949. But there are other long-standing divisions. Circumcision, for example, is a non-starter with the vast majority of the Indian population. As one health worker succinctly put it: 'Hindus are not going to get circumcised and Muslims are already circumcised.'

On other sexual matters, however, there is widespread agreement between the religious groups. Neither the leaders of the Hindus nor the Muslims would take the lead in seeking a radical solution to help the position of sex workers. Nor is there much support for such a policy among the general public. There is a widespread contempt for women who, for whatever reason, have fallen into sex work, but there is also a residual male contempt for the rights of women generally. Charges of exploitation and police corruption fall on deaf ears. Traditionally, Indian women occupy a subservient position. You only have to go to a mixed-gender meeting to see the women respectfully occupying the rear rows. One sympathetic worker in the area set out to me how *he* saw the traditional position: 'A woman is not supposed to be macho. She is not supposed to be sexy. A woman is meant to be submissive. She is not supposed to have power.' More and more of the younger generations, of course, do not accept this for a moment, but some measure of the distance still to go is shown by the recent spate of attacks on women in Delhi. It is at least some measure of progress that such attacks are now reported in both the national and international press, when once they would have been all but ignored.

Nevertheless, the old attitudes persist and from the point of HIV this has a very direct consequence. Out of the 2.1 million people in India living with HIV the government estimates that over 500,000 are undiagnosed. Many of these are women and even when they do test that can come very late – dangerously late – for treatment. In the vast majority of cases, the women will have been infected by their husbands or other male partners but in the eyes of their families that does not absolve them. According to one worker in a charity trying to protect the position of mothers, 'The family blame her for getting the infection. She did something.' If the man dies then the prospect is that the woman will be forced to leave the home – there are many widows living as single women in Delhi. Inside the public health system women with HIV are often treated as second-class citizens, disdained by the doctors and segregated from the other patients. As one woman remarked to me, it is a form of apartheid. In the private sector those living with HIV can be asked to pay more on the grounds that 'we have to throw away the instruments afterwards'. Against such a background it is not surprising that many women do not come forward for testing or put off the day for as long as they can – by which time it is often too late.

It is for reasons like this that men who have sex with men are also reluctant to come forward. According to some I spoke to in Delhi, their position is even lower down the scale of public acceptance than transgender people. It is the familiar story: ostracism for gay men and lesbians, family disgrace, particularly in rural communities, and violence directed against them. Worse still, such hatred was for many long years sanctified by a law which had been passed by the British in 1860 when Lord Canning, who had served in the governments of Peel and Melbourne, was Governor General. The law (section 377 of the Indian penal code) prohibited 'carnal intercourse against the order of nature with any man, woman or animal' and laid down sentences of up to life imprisonment.

Then in 2009 everything changed – or so it seemed. The Delhi High Court lifted section 377 for consenting adults, effectively decriminalising homosexuality. In a memorable phrase the court held that 'discrimination is the antithesis of equality and it is the recognition of equality which will foster the dignity of every individual'. Of course the ruling did not mean that immediately the clouds of prejudice lifted. It was also unclear just how far the writ of the Delhi court ran. But at the very least it meant that a significant step had been taken towards acceptance. It looked as if a nail had been driven through the heart of a very Victorian law. In fact, the law had fallen into disuse and only existed as a threat hanging over the heads of gays and lesbians and to be used to advantage by police prepared to exploit it. If any law should have been pensioned off it was this.

Then, a month after my visit to India, the position changed again. An appeal had been lodged in the Supreme Court and, on his last day in court before his retirement in December 2013, one of the two judges, G. S. Singhvi, ruled that only Parliament could repeal the 1860 British law. So, ironically, in the year that Britain itself moved on to allowing equal marriage, India appeared intent on marooning itself in a bygone age. The gay community was outraged. One of their most influential supporters was Vikram Seth, the author of *A Suitable Boy*, who appeared on the front page of the magazine *India Today* holding a large notice saying 'Not a Criminal'.

In an interview with BBC India he said, 'A judgment which takes away the liberties of at least fifty million gay, bisexual and transgender people in India is scandalous. It is inhumane – and if you wish you can remove the "e" at the end of that word.' As for posing for the magazine photograph (described in the press as an 'unprecedented' action) Mr Seth replied, 'There's nothing heroic in what I have done. There are gay people who live lives of quiet desperation in India's towns and villages. They need people to voice their dismay and disappointments.'

Predictably, this was not the view of the religious leaders. In a remarkable show of unity, they put aside their usual quarrels to back the Supreme Court judgment. One religious leader said, 'This is the right decision. We welcome it. Homosexuality is against Indian culture, against nature and against science.' Another called homosexuality 'a bad addiction' which could be cured. A third said bluntly that 'homosexuality is a crime according to scriptures and is unnatural'. There was even a suggestion that banning homosexuality would help in the fight against HIV and Aids – when all the evidence (together with common sense) suggests the opposite is the case. Making homosexuality a criminal offence simply puts up a massive barrier to testing and treatment.

Caught in this crossfire, it would have been easy for the government of India to have postponed any decision until after the 2014 election and indeed that was the immediate forecast of what their tactics would be. But, to their credit, instead they petitioned the Supreme Court on the basis that the ruling 'violated the principle of equality'. The law minister, Kapil Sibal, said 'let's hope the rights to personal choices is preserved', while the President of the ruling Congress Party, Sonia Gandhi, described the Victorian statute as 'an archaic, unjust law'.

That, however, was not the end of the matter. In January 2014 the Supreme Court rejected the petitions and effectively put the decision back to the government. New legislation seems now to be the only way forward, but that is by no means certain. The main opposition to the Congress Party comes from the Bharatiya Janata Party (BJP) whose roots are in the deeply conservative Hindu religious and cultural organisations and who support the reinstatement of the legal ban. Any attempt to legislate will be deeply controversial, and irrespective of the eventual outcome, the case has confirmed one truth about India – that this vast country contains a very substantial homophobic population. True equality is a distant prospect and without it the battle against HIV and Aids will always be shackled.

The sadness is that there is so much that India has got right. In particular it is a nation that explicitly puts prevention first. What other nation would boldly state that 'prevention has been and will continue to be [our] primary response to the HIV epidemic'? That is certainly not the message that comes from Moscow or Kampala, but nor is it the message from Washington or London. To these nations, prevention is too difficult to measure, too uncertain in a competition for funds. They know what should be spent on treating those who are infected but are unable to make the jump on what to do to prevent infection. India deserves the utmost credit for its efforts in this regard, as do those early decision-makers who set up the National Aids Control Organisation and prevented Aids becoming an out-of-control crisis in India.

Yet in spite of this brave action it is difficult for an outsider like me to see India as a model for the rest of the world. You cannot have as a model a nation where the divisions of the caste system still throw a long shadow of discrimination and prejudice. You cannot have a model where that same prejudice extends to the very priority groups you are trying to reach and where transgender people and many others are treated with such contempt. You cannot have as a model a country where the argument still continues to rage over a 150-year-old law which criminalises homosexuals, which discourages testing and treatment, and gives cover for the views of bigots.

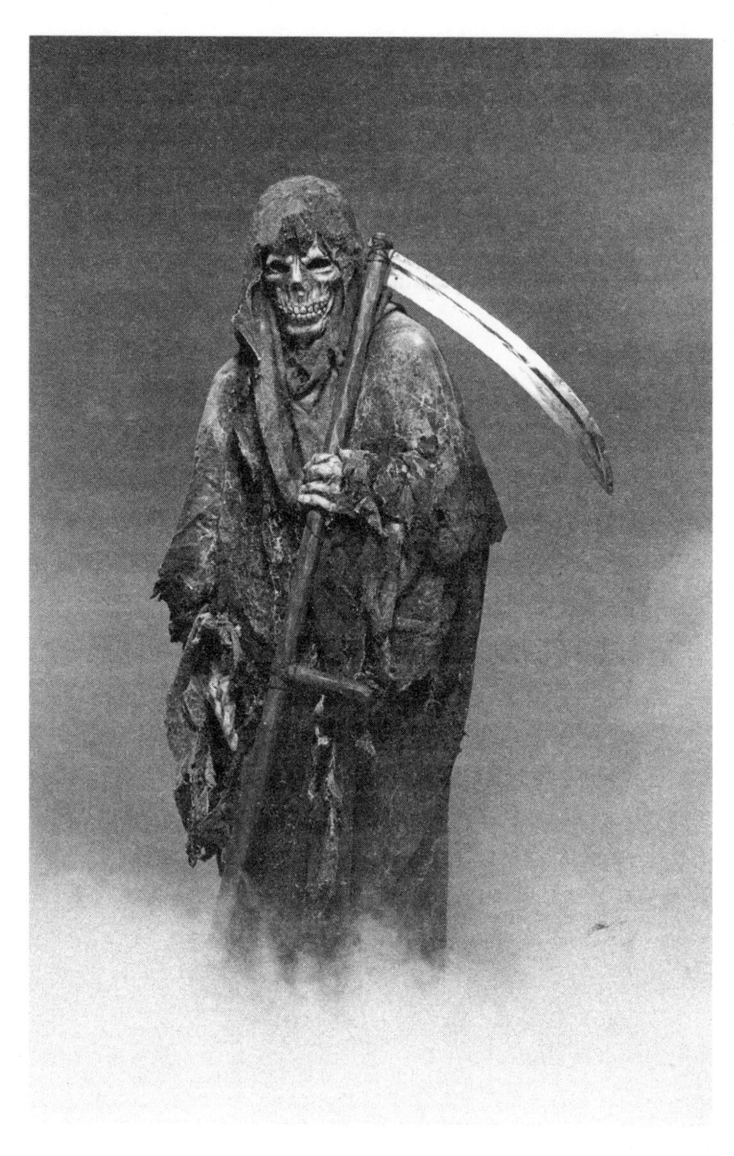

The controversial but successful 'Grim Reaper' advertisement of the late 1980s, warning the Australian public of the dangers of Aids.

NINE

SYDNEY: THE PROMISED LAND?

NOVEMBER, AND THE jacaranda trees are in full purple and in the city's gardens the canna shine out a fresh, bright scarlet. On the quay crowds gather around the signature sails of the Opera House and if you look up to the iron girders of the massive Harbour Bridge you can see a small line of tiny specks being led in a human chain across the top span. In the harbour ferry boats criss-cross the water and a group of white sailing yachts change tack to catch the wind. This is Sydney, New South Wales. It is home to about a quarter of Australia's twenty-two million population, and it has prospered and has survived better than most during the international financial crisis. It is a city of business with a skyline dominated by the tall, oblongs of concrete and glass which house the banks and the insurance companies. It is also a city of galleries, music and theatre. But for our purposes, it is a city where some say policies towards HIV are the best in the world. So is this the promised land?

A few miles from the centre of Sydney there is a small block of offices by the side of a quiet square with a war memorial to the dozens of young men from Redfern who perished in two world wars. The well-kept building contains the smart offices of the Scarlet Alliance, which represents Australian sex workers. The alliance was formed back in 1989 in an effort to afford some protection against exploitation. Today, after a remarkable set of reforms, sex work in New South Wales is entirely legal and basically run just like any other business. Brothels must meet normal business requirements but here there is no question of them or the sex workers being specially licensed. The protection comes from standard occupational health and safety laws. Brothels, strip clubs, massage parlours, escort services and street prostitution are all now within the law. Street workers in Sydney can take their clients to 'safe houses' – with security on the gate – and so avoid the violence which is the occupational hazard of the sex worker's life. There is none of the hypocrisy of so many nations that prostitutes should be allowed but not seen.

Janelle Fawkes, the chief executive of the alliance, is a softly spoken woman who, like all her executive committee, was once a sex worker herself. She says the effect of the new laws, which were introduced in the mid-1990s, has been entirely beneficial both to sex workers and to the public generally. There is not the corruption that typified the previous free-for-all. Although it would be an exaggeration to say there are no complaints, they mainly come today not on moral grounds but on planning grounds from people who do not want to live next door to a brothel. Most crucial in the terms of this book, Janelle Fawkes claims that the record in public health terms is outstanding. HIV rates among sex workers are less than 1 per cent. Rates of sexually transmitted infections are also very low. There is no recent case of HIV being passed on by a sex worker and the use of condoms is virtually 100 per cent. It seems to be the kind of outcome that nations around the world have been seeking.

So how was this deeply pragmatic policy, which seems to ride roughshod over the usual opposition of politicians and Church, introduced? It goes back to the Royal Commission on the Police which between 1995 and 1997 examined corruption inside the New South Wales force to devastating effect. In page after page it exposed an almost incredibly long list of abuses, including police perjury, the planting of evidence, theft and extortion, interference with internal investigations, the police code of silence – and police protection of club and vice operators. They found that brothel managers were paying protection money to the police and that, in one area, local brothels were providing police with free alcohol and sexual services. The commission's investigation was so detailed and comprehensive that it could not be ignored. Dozens of police left the service. They took advantage of an amnesty against prosecution, were dismissed or retired. Others were prosecuted and several committed suicide once the extent of the corruption was revealed.

The New South Wales government had a choice – the kind of choice which other countries throughout the world have faced and still face. They could have denounced the sex work and tried to legislate it out of existence, or they could have tried to brush it under the carpet and hope it could be kept out of sight. In the event they faced up to the issue and, in the words of the commission, they allowed well-run brothels to operate on the basis that 'a potential opportunity for corrupt conduct on the part of the police was closed off'. There was a lengthy and fierce debate in both houses of the New South Wales Parliament but, in the end, the legislation was passed as a bipartisan measure.

So just how well has this radically reformed system worked out? In 2012 the Kirby Institute at the University of New South Wales, in cooperation with Melbourne University, published a study of the position in three Australian cities: Sydney, where sex work has been largely decriminalised; Melbourne, where brothels or individual sex workers must be licensed; and Perth where most forms of commercial sex are illegal but where there is a limited licensing scheme. There was no question which city came out best. They found that New South Wales had 'one of the healthiest sex industries ever documented'.

The report confirmed the claims of the Scarlet Alliance. Condom use in Sydney brothels was virtually 100 per cent and the prevalence of other sexually transmitted diseases was at least as good as the general population and probably better. Contrary to original fears, decriminalisation had not led to an increase in numbers of sex workers. The number of sex workers in Sydney brothels was similar to twenty years previously, when the new system was introduced.

As for the alternative models found in Melbourne and Perth, the report was damning. Licensing, which on the face of it sounds an attractive halfway house, came in for particular criticism. Professor Basil Donovan from the Kirby Institute said, 'Jurisdictions that try to ban or license sex work always lose track as most of the industry slides into the shadows.' In Queensland, 90 per cent of the sex industry was operating illegally and in Victoria the figure was 50 per cent. The report said, 'Licensing systems are expensive and difficult to administer and they always generate an unlicensed underclass. That underclass is wary of and avoids surveillance systems and public health services ... licensing is a threat to public health.' In Sydney there are also some sex workers operating outside the regulations, but the problem is not remotely on the same scale as with licensing.

The report also provided a sketch of the sex workers and their clients. Compared to their counterparts in Perth and Melbourne, the brothel-based sex workers in Sydney were better educated and, although they were more likely to have been born in an Asian or other non-English-speaking country, there was virtually no evidence of trafficking or coercion. Indeed, the position was a substantial improvement on the pre-reform position when sex workers in brothels were typically poorly educated women from Thailand, with false passports and visas, and usually in debt to the agents who had organised their travel to Australia. As for men, only 2.3 per cent of men in New South Wales purchased sexual services in any one year.

The finding of the report was that reform in Sydney had 'improved human rights; removed police corruption; netted savings for the criminal justice system; and enhanced the surveillance, health promotion, and safety of the New South Wales sex industry'. To which I would add that the sex workers I met in Delhi, Kiev and Washington would all have dearly loved such a system.

None of this of course will still the international debate. Everyone has a view and politicians are likely to head for what they see as the popular ground. The absolutist position is that selling sex is just wrong and therefore sex work should be banned altogether. The trouble with this argument is that over the ages it has failed as a practical solution. Sex work has continued but it has simply gone underground, with the obvious effects that proper health checks have been ignored and criminality encouraged. That is why in most nations we have reached not prohibition but a no man's land of disapproving acceptance. There is no great morality in allowing the resulting exploitation and corruption, but that is what most of the world prefers to do. As is the case in India, we allow the pimps to prosper at the expense of the sex workers and the gangsters to grease the palms of the police while we look the other way.

A variation on prohibition is to make it illegal for clients to *buy* sex, but to abolish the crime of soliciting and, at the same time, to set up schemes to help sex workers leave the trade. In February 2014 the *Times* columnist Janice Turner came out in support of such schemes, saying that 'across Europe the mood has changed' and pointing to efforts in France and the European Parliament to go down this road. The article produced a swift rejoinder from some of those working in the area. Further criminalising sex work, they argued, would have serious adverse effects whether or not it was focused on the buyer or the seller. It would not stop people selling sex but would drive sex work underground. The group added, 'It would also enforce stigma through legislation and this will make it far less likely for sex workers to engage with sexual health and social care services and report to the police if they are attacked.'

If I were a citizen of Sydney in this debate I would say that here we have a system which works. We have reduced sexual disease and virtually eliminated sex workers passing on HIV. Sensible precautions like the use of condoms are very widely followed and police corruption has been eliminated. Violence against sex workers has been substantially reduced and the amount of sex work outside the law is limited. If I lived in Sydney I would also say, 'You show me how any new system would improve on that and, also incidentally, if this is to be a worldwide policy, just how you intend to help sex workers find alternative work in Africa and India.' Treating sex work as a normal business may not be the perfect solution. Different surveys in different countries show that many sex workers feel exploited and would like to leave the occupation. The trouble is that driving sex work underground does not prevent exploitation – it encourages it – and at the same time endangers both public health and the health of the sex worker. Sensible control may be as far as we can get today and for the foreseeable future. As for criminalisation, the internet and mobile phones make the law extremely difficult to enforce and mean that predominantly it is the street workers who are prosecuted. Business controls at least hold out the prospect for sex workers that they escape the miserable subservience and violence that characterises their lives in so many countries today, while also providing a substantial step forward in public health.

When the New South Wales Royal Commission presented its final report in 1997, sex work was not the only activity that came under scrutiny. Their most critical findings centred on the police and illegal drugs, particularly in the Kings Cross area, which has always been the centre of the drugs trade in Sydney. The commission found that there was:

> *An overwhelming body of evidence suggesting the existence of close relationships between police and those*

> *involved in the supply of drugs. This encompassed a variety of activities ranging from police turning a blind eye to the criminality of the favoured in return for regular payments; to active assistance when they happened to be caught; to tip-offs of pending police activity; and to affirmative police action aimed at driving out competitors.*

In Kings Cross itself there were 'shooting galleries' permitted by the police on the basis that medical assistance would be on hand for those who overdosed. The trouble was that supervision was left in the hands of people who lacked any medical training, had criminal records, and were closely involved in the supply of drugs. The arrangements placed no emphasis on rehabilitation, and referral to the public health system was clearly against the interests of those running the 'galleries'.

Today the position is very different. Standing on the outskirts of Kings Cross, a short taxi ride from the sex workers' headquarters in Redfern, is the old Darlinghurst fire station. Today it houses the Kirketon Road Centre where drug users can come to collect their methadone and clean needles and where there is a room where injecting can be medically supervised. To reach it you pass two vending machines at the building's entrance offering a clean needle and syringe for two Australian dollars and follow an uncovered, narrow staircase up to the crowded waiting room.

The director of the centre, whom I met on my visit in November 2012, is the vivacious Dr Ingrid van Beek who also works in under-developed countries overseas with the Global Fund. She told me that the result of adopting a clean-needle policy is that today the number of injecting drug users who contract HIV is 'minuscule'. 'The time for governments who have not yet introduced the policy to talk of pilot schemes is past,' she added. 'We know what works.' She readily concedes, however, that it is easier to do in countries with developed health care systems than it is in countries which do not even have the facilities for prenatal work.

Today there are around 1,000 needle and syringe outlets in New South Wales including pharmacies, and automatic machines which dispense boxes of six needles. The centre runs a bus that takes the harm-reduction message (together with needles, condoms and testing kits) throughout the Kings Cross district. Everyone is refreshingly open about the problem. In the 1990s used needles and syringes littered the streets. Today there are collecting bins – even on the ferry to the popular beach at Manly.

Reviewing the success of the clean-needle policy Dr van Beek shares the views of clinicians and police in other countries – that there is absolutely no evidence of increased criminality as a result of this policy. She says that the evidence is not of more crime, but of drug users being reached by the health service for the first time: 'Thirty years ago people who injected would not have been anywhere near the health service.' Her personal view is that, as a general policy, the use of drugs should be decriminalised but the efforts should be maintained to counter the importers and the pushers.

As for methadone, she says: 'Methadone produces a transformation in a user's lifestyle and that is obviously good. But down the track you face problems of quality of life. Your life is limited by when you can get your methadone. So if you can come off it altogether then that is obviously good.' But she warns that compulsory targets will not work. Each case needs to be managed – one to one. It is the antidote to the view of some politicians that users can be forced off methadone in a set time and easy public spending savings achieved. If only it were so.

Sydney still remains a centre for drugs, although drug use itself has changed. In the 1990s there was a glut of cheap heroin imported from the golden triangle of Thailand, Burma and Laos with the result that the number of users injecting drugs increased. Then in 2001 there was a dramatic reduction in supply. No one quite knows why, but the most popular theory is that the suppliers found easier markets at home and in China and Indonesia. The price was not so high but it was easier to distribute and there was a much bigger market. One result in Sydney has been that as supply has decreased, the price of heroin has increased and the number of injectors has reduced. One doctor told me, 'The average age of injectors is around thirty. Young people are not taking it up. It is too expensive.'

So both in sex work and drug taking there has been a substantial revolution in Sydney, much of which can be put down to the work and revelations of the 1997 Royal Commission. It is perhaps here that there is a lesson for the rest of the world. The inquiries revealed precisely the problems that New South Wales faced. The corruption which they established was of long standing, but it was only when it was exposed in detail that politicians took the kind of measures that were necessary. It was the catalyst for change. The approach was broadly bipartisan and based on evidence. Many of the old prejudices were forgotten in the name of better public health and the end of corruption. What would be the effect if similar commissions of inquiry were to look at the position in Moscow or Delhi – or for that matter Washington or London?

Sydney has not always been so advanced. Back in the 1980s Bill Bowtell was chief adviser to the federal health minister, Neal Blewett, in the very early days of the HIV epidemic in Australia. 'It was a horrible period,' he told me. 'People were scared. Some said it was the judgement of God and that Aids was something that killed sinners.' Cars were burnt because people who had been in them had HIV. Nurses pushed food under the door to Aids patients. Sitting in a small café in the shadow of Sydney's St Vincent's Hospital, he also remembers that clean-needle exchanges were opposed by many, including doctors, on the grounds that it would lead to more crime. 'If crime goes up we will come after you,' the Australian Medical Association told him encouragingly. Are doctors' unions the same the world over?

This was of course the time when there were no antiretroviral drugs and public education was the only option. Blewett and the Hawke government decided on a very similar approach to what we were doing in Britain. Indeed Sammy Harari, who oversaw much of the British advertising, also worked in Australia. In the resulting campaign, rather than being presented with gravestones and white lilies, the public in Australia were warned by the grim reaper, scythe in hand, ready to cut down anyone who did not take sensible precautions. Today when journalists look back at these campaigns they tend to refer to both Britain's tombstone and Australia's grim reaper as 'notorious', ignoring the fact that in both countries HIV and other sexual diseases fell sharply. As Bowtell says, 'It was the only weapon we had. People were dying.' Today such a campaign would be strangled by a focus group but, of course, the difference is that we now have the drugs to preserve life. The real criticism is that no one has had the wit (or the money) to develop an effective campaign for the second decade of the twenty-first century.

New South Wales, if not the rest of the nation, has travelled a vast distance since those early days. Politicians and health professionals in Sydney take a pride in the city's reputation. The approach has been bipartisan, pragmatic and down to earth. The guiding principle is: 'We do what it takes.' Successive ministers of health in New South Wales have shown a commitment to HIV absent in other countries and have not been afraid of challenging the orthodox. Sydney has led the way, but there are others who are not afraid of new ideas. When I was there in 2012, the prison authorities in Canberra were exploring the idea of a clean-needle scheme in prison on the basis that everything should be done to avoid prisoners sharing. The argument was that, as everyone knew that drugs were used in prisons the world over, you could provide clean needles in just the same way as condoms were provided for protection in prisoner sex.

Another feature of the Australian approach at its best is how public health authorities have worked in partnership with the organisations representing the people who have contracted HIV. One official told me:

> *In the early days we could not have done it without the cooperation of the infected communities. HIV drew governments into areas where they didn't want to go. Financing the injecting of drugs was not something that governments expected to do. But it became quite clear that the traditional model of 'the war against drugs' had failed. The aim became to prevent others being put at risk.*

So is this as good as it gets? It may well be that it is, but that does not mean that the position either in Sydney or in Australia generally is ideal. In Australia there are about 32,000 people living with HIV with around 8,000 unaware of their condition and undiagnosed. What gives most cause for concern – and the charge that Australia has lost momentum – is the relentless rise in the number of new infections. These are tracked by the Kirby Institute in Sydney and the latest figures show that nationally in 2012 there was a 10 per cent increase in cases to 1,253 – the biggest rise in the annual figures for two decades. Back in 1999 the total was 724 new diagnoses. The New South Wales figures are the worst in the whole country.

As in virtually every country I have visited around the world, all the public health officials say the urgent need is for more testing. But here there is a failure in the Australian system. To take a test is a cumbersome process. You go in, wait and pay but it is not until a week later that you get the result – and then you are invited to come in again, wait and pay. The doctors and the laboratories stand in the way of speeding up the process and home testing seems a long way distant. It is a system-wide failure according to an editor based in Sydney:

It's the same for any other test, and it's a real pain. Basically they won't give results by post or phone, which of course also sucks up the doctor's time. You also can't get repeat prescriptions without paying to see the doctor every time, and one prescription will only provide six months' therapy. So you have to go back. And wait. And pay – pretty much so the doctor can just push the print button on the computer. I would be willing to bet that would lead to people coming off HIV treatment.

The HIV position in both Australia and New South Wales is dominated by men having sex with men. Around two-thirds of new diagnoses nationally are of gay men and the reasons for the rise in infections are not too difficult to find. About a third of gay men admit to having unprotected sex. Many will never have even seen the 'grim reaper' advertisements of the 1980s but, even more ominously, according to Professor Andrew Grulich of the Kirby Institute, 'the fear has fallen away even among those who remember the early days'. There is now a false complacence typical of many other countries where there is easy access to antiretroviral drugs. There may not be a cure, they seem to think, but surely all that is needed is a pill a day. It is the other side of the treatment coin and ignores all the problems – mental as well as physical – that go with HIV. Personally, I have never met anyone with HIV who laughs it off as a trivial inconvenience. A useful part of public education would be to spell out the consequences.

Better sex education in schools would also help. In Sydney it is left to the principals of the schools to determine. Some do it well, including some (but not all) Catholic schools. Others are seriously wanting. One local health worker told me that 'In many schools it is not addressed at all – or if addressed it is guided by the moral view of the teacher or the school. It is not objective health advice. Yet if you ask parents if they favour sex and relationship lessons there is overwhelming support.'

Sadly there seems a real risk that rather than improving the position, it may become worse. In January 2014 a two-man team was appointed to review the national school curriculum. One of the two, Kevin Donnelly, has decided views on what relationship and sex education in schools should contain. In a book he wrote in 2004, he argued that many parents believed that the sex education in schools should be strictly limited. He wrote: 'Many parents would consider the sexual practices of gays, lesbians and transgender individuals decidedly unnatural and that such groups have a greater risk in terms of transmitting sexual diseases and Aids.'

You could of course argue that the lack of good sex education lies behind the big increases in other sexually transmitted diseases, particularly among younger people. New notifications of chlamydia in 2011 reached almost 80,000; the numbers have tripled over the last decade. The most affected were women between fifteen and twenty-four. Gonorrhoea has also increased sharply in the last ten years with almost 12,000 new cases a year mainly affecting young men. The public health message is failing to get through to young people.

And what about the prejudice against gay people so prevalent in many other countries and which has such a devastating impact on the willingness to test? I have yet to come across a country where there is no prejudice. Not one.

We should remember also that Australia was one of the last major countries to decriminalise homosexuality. Ending the British colonial laws established after 1788 was a long, tortuous business. New South Wales did not get around to it until 1989 and the very last state to decriminalise was Tasmania in 1997. We should not assume that even today acceptance is enthusiastically embraced by everyone, even in a liberal city like Sydney. As it happens, Australia has now been presented with what many gay people would regard as a test case, although others would regard it as more a test of religious belief.

In October 2013 the legislative assembly of the Australian Capital Territory (ACT), with a population of almost 400,000, passed a law which made equal marriage legal in Canberra – or so they thought. The effect was that for five days same-sex couples could get married in Australia's capital city and twenty-seven couples did just that. However, in mid-December 2013, the Australian High Court intervened and ruled that the Federal Marriage Act, which was amended by Prime Minister John Howard in 2004 to stipulate that marriage could only be between a man and a woman, took precedence over any state and territory legislation. The only way that the law could be changed was (as we saw in India with the legalisation of homosexuality itself) by an act of federal parliament.

The question now is whether the Conservative Australian Prime Minister Tony Abbott, who came to office in September 2013, will follow David Cameron, the

Conservative Prime Minister in London, and change the national law. The prospect does not look promising. It was after all the federal government that successfully challenged the ruling of the ACT court but, more importantly, Abbott himself is a stern opponent of same-sex marriage. He also realises the political implication of any move to reform the position. No more than in Britain is it a vote winning issue for a Conservative leader with his own party. The only reason to legislate in London in 2013 was because it was right – and that was the view of both Houses of Parliament on a free vote. The solution in Australia could be to follow that example and allow a free vote if ever an equal marriage bill is introduced. My own view is that in the end the reformers will win here and the question is not whether but when. It will be a vast pity if a country like Australia, which has set the pace in so many ways, failed this test.

To my mind Sydney is at the same time the most relaxed and the most sensible city I visited. In dealing with HIV the leaders here have been both pragmatic and successful. But those working in the field are slightly aghast at the prospect of Sydney being set up as the promised land. 'It is at that point that complacency sets in,' one doctor said to me. Nevertheless, in terms of prevention and treatment there are few cities that can match it. Certainly Sydney can teach the cities of Europe and the Old World a few lessons.

GIRLS SAVE SOHO
Women of colour Say NO EVICTIONS Safety First!
I'd rather sell my body in Soho than sell my mind to a corporation!
Save the Girls Save Soho
epay

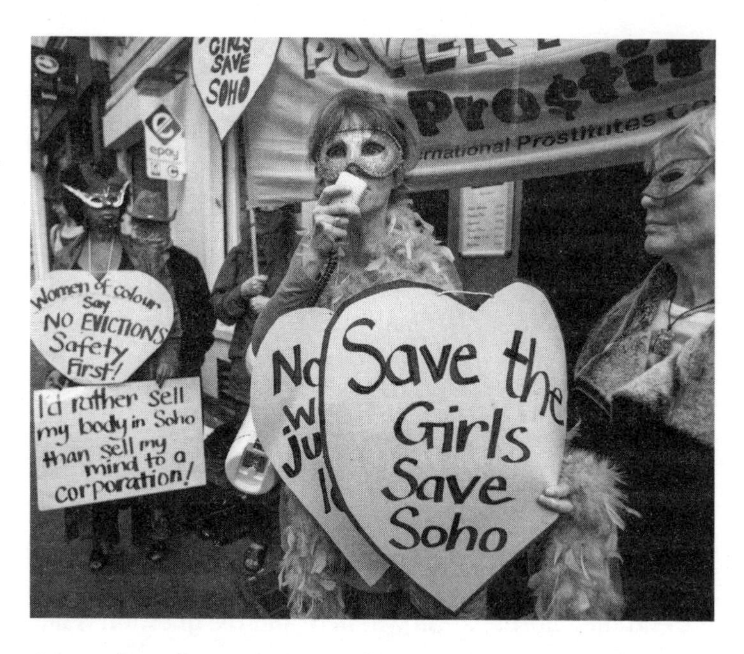

Sex workers demonstrate against attempts to evict them from Soho in 2014.

TEN

LONDON: IS IT STILL A PROBLEM?

AS LIONEL BART might have said, 'fings ain't what they used to be'. In Soho there have always been drugs on sale if you knew where to go. Twenty-five years ago it was the traditional illegal selection of heroin, cocaine, ecstasy and, of course, cannabis. Today a new variety is up for sale, and by their very nature they pose a new threat. These are the 'ChemSex' drugs, which have the effect of prolonging sex, removing inhibitions and all too often leading to unprotected sex. They consist of methamphetamine (crystal meth) and mephedrone, as well as a number of other drugs like GBL. According to one survey, many of the drug users are HIV positive, many share needles to inject the drugs, and many have several sexual partners during a weekend of drug use. In short, ChemSex drugs can be a sure way to spread HIV.

The ChemSex drugs all have the same effect; the difference between them is price. The most expensive is crystal meth at about £250 a gram while mephedrone at £30 a gram is regarded as the poor man's substitute. A few years ago the experts were saying that crystal meth did not pose a threat in Britain, but in 2007 it was reclassified as a Class A drug – in the top league of British illegality. But according to those working in the field the ban has made little difference to supply and both drugs are 'readily available'.

There is no doubt who are the predominant users in Britain: men who have sex with men. And with the new drugs have come a new kind of injector. David Stuart, Substance Use Adviser at the Soho Sexual Health Clinic, told me:

> *The heroin users out on the streets know how to inject and keep safe. It is one of the successes of the clean-needles policy. The new injectors are blindingly ignorant but it is more than that. Eighty per cent of men who have sex with men don't inject themselves in any event. Someone else does it for them. The heroin user gets a high. They want to escape. With gay men it is something else altogether. It is about sex but most of all it is about connecting.*

Men who have sex with men are today the chief source of HIV in London, and Soho is one of the undoubted centres for what some say has become the gay capital of Europe.

It is not that gay people live in the narrow streets between London's theatre land on Shaftesbury Avenue and the big stores of Oxford Street but Soho is a place where they can meet and drink – and drink. There are said to be fifty gay clubs and pubs in a 500-metre radius of Dean Street. You only have to walk in the streets on a Saturday night past the crowds spilling onto the pavement to see Soho's popularity. But it is not the only gay centre in London. Just south of the Thames is the 'Vauxhall gay village', complete with clubs and saunas. In the autumn of 2012 two gay men died after overdosing in a sauna and there are persistent stories of ambulances each week taking three or four drug users away for emergency treatment at the nearby St Thomas' hospital. Dr John White, a consultant at the hospital, confirms that 'new drugs are coming along all the time' and also confirms the danger of a highly addictive drug like crystal meth. 'One month they have a good job,' he says. 'A few weeks later they have fallen apart. It's very rapid. They get captured.'

The truth is, however, that today you need neither clubs nor saunas. The internet age is transforming the position. Private parties are arranged in flats – not so much in the public housing in the heart of Lambeth but in the smart £1 million-plus flats nearer the river and conveniently placed for the offices of the City or the West End. HIV has always included the affluent as the celebrity deaths down the years have proved. The middle-class drug users are doubtless living next door to the very people who so commonly today ask about HIV: 'You don't hear much about it these days. Is it still a problem?'

The internet today provides new opportunities for men to get together which did not exist twenty-five years ago. There is a proliferation of online sites and mobile apps used by gay men to find sex partners. With a few clicks on a smartphone or site you can find photographs of a large selection of men, ready, willing and also near. Just to avoid confusion, adverts come complete with tags like a dollar sign to indicate a sex worker, or 'BB' to indicate bareback, or unprotected, sex. Connecting with casual sexual partners is easier than ever; the trouble is that in connecting they often forget (if they were ever taught) about the dangers of shared needles.

At this stage I should make one point absolutely clear. The position I describe is not typical of the lives of gay people generally. I remember one gay man saying to me that if only the public knew how 'ordinary' so many gay lives were, there would not be so much emotion generated. He had been with his partner for over fifteen years, was in a civil partnership and wanted now to marry. He said: 'The great thing is that in the evening you can come home and talk about the stresses of the day.' Just like any other couple. Nor are ChemSex drugs a feature of huge numbers of gay men's lives. Paul Steinbeck, a prevention expert working in Lambeth, says: 'It is not the case that everybody is doing it. It is a significant problem for a small number of gay men.'

The point is that ChemSex drugs symbolise the new challenges that are forever arising. When I mounted my Aids campaign in 1986 the internet had hardly been invented and the smartphone was still to come. Since then all experience has shown that you ignore new developments in HIV at your peril and it is better to overreact than ignore. In the case of the ChemSex drugs there is no inherent reason why their use should be confined to gay men, and the dangers of risky sexual practices are no different from the ones I warned about thirty years ago.

For decades Britain has become accustomed to minuscule figures for HIV caused by shared needles. Clean needles and methadone remain the foundation of policy, but policies that have worked well for the traditional group targeted by clean-needle schemes – injecting heroin users – will not necessarily be as effective for the middle-class ChemSex users sharing needles and having sexual marathons in the privacy of their Vauxhall flats. As one doctor said, 'You won't cope just by a van at the side of the road dispensing condoms and needles.' It is just as well, then, that we are seeing today the emergence in London of a new breed of sexual health clinics.

For decades sexual health has been a 'Cinderella' subject inside the health service. For years the clinics' services were not even named as sexual health, but labelled under the deeply unappealing banner of Genito-Urinary Medicine (GUM). Too often the clinic was placed in the most inaccessible and unattractive part of the hospital. One consultant who moved to Soho said that he came from a hospital where the clinic was in the basement – and that to reach it you went past the mortuary. Today that is changing. You can hardly believe that the clinic at 56 Dean Street, with its bright and imaginative design, is part of the National Health Service which, for all its merits, has never been accused of being stylish. The same can be said of the purpose-built clinic in Burrell Street, just south of Blackfriars Bridge in Lambeth's neighbouring borough, Southwark. At the Homerton University Hospital at Hackney in East London, the clinic may still be at the rear of the hospital but the newly opened Jonathan Mann centre has transformed the public offering. Rather than being viewed from outside as places of blame and shame, London's sexual health clinics are now being seen much more as places for treatment *and* advice.

And there is no doubt that advice is needed. At Dean Street, David Stuart says that some of young men who come in are isolated and unsure about their sexuality. 'The task is to take them from promiscuity to a relationship,' he says. 'You can enjoy sex but there are alternatives to the bar and club scene.' Another belief that needs to be punctured is that there is no great drawback to HIV these days. The obvious warning of what one doctor called 'the walking skeletons and the dying' has disappeared. The dangerous new belief is that all that is needed these days is one daily pill.

Countering this Professor Jane Anderson at Homerton, who is one of the most committed clinicians in the country, says:

HIV remains an incurable, stigmatising condition that requires lifelong treatment. It burrows both into people's cells and into their identities. It changes people's relationships with themselves and those around them. It cuts people off from one another, it interrupts intimacy and compromises self-worth and self-belief. People tell me that after a diagnosis of HIV they feel fearful, worthless, isolated. The most up-to-date clinical expertise alone cannot solve the complex problems that HIV presents.

The first need, in London as elsewhere in Britain and the rest of the world, is for more effective testing and it is this which the clinics are trying to provide. The Dean Street clinic has taken the tests into the gay bars with surprisingly good results in persuading men who have never tested before. At the clinic itself, tests can be done very quickly and the results confirmed within thirty minutes. The Burrell Street clinic operates a seven-day-a-week service, with the result that at a weekend the clinic can see 200 patients, with people waiting at the door when the doctors arrive in the morning. Such efforts and more are needed throughout London. Late diagnoses (leading to late treatment) remain responsible for the bulk of Aids-related deaths.

According to a 2013 paper commissioned by the directors of public health in London, about one in five Londoners living with HIV is undiagnosed, but they are responsible for over half of all new HIV infections in the capital. So unless you tackle the issue of the people who are not aware that they are HIV positive, the position continues to deteriorate. You need a policy that will bring in not just the men having sex with men but also the Black African and Black Caribbean populations (where most cases are heterosexually acquired), many of whom live south of the river in Lambeth and Southwark. Together they make up the second largest group affected and also pose some familiar problems.

One of them is stigma. According to one consultant in Southwark it is one of the main reasons why persuading people to test can be so difficult:

> *There is a huge amount of stigma in the Black African population. The fear is that a positive test finding will leak out and the impact that will have in the local community. They can be vilified. If one person finds out he can text it out to all his friends.*

He could, of course, be speaking in Entebbe. There is only one fear greater than being known to be HIV positive and that is to be identified as a man who has sex with other men.

It is almost a relief to turn from the complexities of the new drug injectors and the seemingly intractable problem of hostility to gay people to the traditional sex workers of Soho and another of the HIV priority groups. Or rather, it is a relief until you discover the complexities and the changes that have taken place here too.

An objective view of those changes comes from Central London Action on Sexual Health (CLASH), an unusual but highly effective part of the health service. It was formed in the late 1980s specifically because of HIV, and specifically to make contact with the hard to reach, high risk groups like sex workers and the homeless as well as men who have sex with men. At that time, these groups certainly did not go near the health service. The first work of CLASH was to provide free condoms and free needles, particularly to the street-based sex workers. Today it has developed to a drop-in centre just on the western edge of Soho, not far from the designer shopping of Regent Street and Savile Row. It has a clinic twice a week and provides advice and treatment. The health position of the sex workers at present is that HIV is 'very unusual' and although there have been increases in chlamydia and gonorrhoea they only match the increases in the general population. Such results are a compliment to CLASH and other organisations like the Terrence Higgins Trust, with which it works closely.

A pen picture of the sex workers who come to CLASH would be this. Most come from Eastern Europe and are between about eighteen and thirty. Most have children and many have partners, although not necessarily with them in Soho. They operate from walk-in flats with their own maids – women who may have been sex workers themselves and who keep an eye on the CCTV to check on the clients coming up the stairs. The cash however goes straight to the sex worker who will almost certainly be paying an exorbitant daily rent for the rooms – up to £350 a day. Even with these outgoings the sex worker makes substantially more money than she would in a bar or serving in a restaurant. The money earned might go home to help her family, or to buy a house, or even to take out private health insurance. Many try not to tell their families about their work and some look back sadly to their previous lives as 'when I was normal'.

According to CLASH the public health danger is that competition among sex workers is fierce. Prices have basically not increased for ten years and unprotected sex is the extra that can be offered for a higher price. As one CLASH worker told me:

> *Everybody is struggling to make a living. Customers want oral sex without a condom and the sex worker is in no position to refuse. If all the women decided together that they would all put up the prices then the customer would have to pay and the women would not be forced to make these concessions. But there's a lot of distrust among the women and agreement is impossible. When the women are asked 'do you do unprotected sex' everyone says no, but they are very happy to point the finger and say who does.*

In its heyday there were perhaps eighty or a hundred flats dotted around Soho used for sex work but over the last few years there has been a drive to close them down. The sex workers say that a deliberate policy is taking place to hand the buildings over for development. Whether that is true or not there is no doubt that at the beginning of 2014 there was a raid involving 200 police many in riot gear and accompanied by dog units. According to Nikki Adams, the spokeswoman for the English Collective of Prostitutes, the sex workers were subjected to 'a very serious and abusive form of policing'. Around forty police forced their way into one flat and one woman was paraded in the street in her underclothes. The press were invited to watch – in spite of the fear that sex workers have of being photographed.

In *The Observer* the actor Rupert Everett who was there at the time of the raid described the scene: 'Flashing police vans blocked the road ... It was an image of war, replete with entrenched photographers and journalists.' More support came from Simon Buckley the vicar of St Anne's in Soho, who protested to the Bishop of London at the action. Personally I would have thought that the Metropolitan Police had enough enemies just now without being portrayed as persecuting women. The result is that almost twenty flats were closed down. Closures like this are a matter for the magistrates' courts and a matter of civil law which does not require that cases are established 'beyond reasonable doubt' as in the criminal law. This is probably just as well for the police. They might have been hard pressed to convince a jury on trafficking and rape which was the apparent reason for the raid.

You may ask, however, whether it is legal in any event for sex workers to operate from flats in the way they have been doing for years past. Chris Higgins of CLASH defines the legal position succinctly: 'All the activities around prostitution are illegal but selling sex is not.' A little more than fifty years ago if you went into Hyde Park from Paddington you passed a line of five or six sex workers touting for business. After a famous report by Sir John Wolfenden in 1957 soliciting for business was eventually banned. So too was advertising for clients including placing cards in telephone booths which used to be obvious and common in London. I noticed however strolling through Soho that it was still possible to put up in neon lights a less than enigmatic notice simply saying 'OPEN' at the entrance to a flat.

I thought in my innocence that although the law might not be entirely clear on soliciting and advertising, at least it should be pretty simple for it to define a brothel. It is not so of course. According to the Crown Prosecution Service, 'The definition of a brothel in English law does not require that the premises are used for the purposes of prostitution since a brothel exists wherever more than one person offers sexual intercourse, whether for payment or not.' I had always thought that the whole basis for legislation was to combat criminally organised prostitution. Apparently not but it explains why sex workers operate from their own rented flats in Soho. Provided that she and her maid do the organising and no one from outside is involved then it is legal. It is also legal if different women work in different flats in the same building provided there is no common organisation. Sex work is the archetypal small business – just banned from growing larger.

At this point I have to confess a certain sympathy for the police creeps in. How on earth are they expected to enforce such a hotch-potch of law and at the same time carry out their essential job, which is to prevent the violence and worse which is all too often the fate of sex workers in London today – and even more so outside the capital. The Home Office funded scheme Ugly Mugs allows sex workers to report attacks anonymously, and *The Guardian* reported that in the twelve months after its launch in July 2012, 400 incidents had been reported. Of those, 106 were sexual assaults and sixty-eight rapes.

I imagine that very few can believe the present legal position is satisfactory. There is no doubt what most sex workers in Soho and elsewhere would want. They would want something like the decriminalised system in New South Wales or in New Zealand (where the law was changed in 2003). Their case is that they sell sex of their own free will. They may have been driven to do so by poverty in their own country, but they deny that trafficking is a major issue. To my mind this all adds up to the need for an absolutely objective inquiry to review the general position of sex work in the capital, including the impact on public health – another Wolfenden inquiry which, as well as changing sex work, paved the way for the eventual decriminalisation of homosexuality – at a time when over 1,000 men were actually serving prison sentences for the 'offence'.

What is needed is an inquiry first to establish what exactly is happening in Britain today. Why is there the violence? How have we had 144 murders (to date) since 1990? What is the evidence for trafficking? What is the evidence for exploitation? A properly independent inquiry would also examine the arguments put forward in favour of the Nordic solution (in which the buyer, not the seller, is prosecuted) backed not only in Sweden and Norway but, at the beginning of 2014, by the European Parliament. It is a solution which recognises the rights of women, but the price is that it creates a new criminal offence which has to be enforced by the long-suffering police. The other fear is that sex work would go underground – and that really would pose a problem for public health.

So is HIV still a problem in Britain and in London? The figures speak for themselves. In 2012 there were 100,000 people in the United Kingdom living with HIV and in that year there were almost 6,400 new diagnoses. Men having sex with men accounted for over half of the new cases and the estimated total of 3,250 was the highest number ever reported. Around a fifth of the people living with HIV remained undiagnosed and during the year there had been 500 deaths – many the result of late diagnosis and the delay in coming forward for testing.

There is no doubt where the problem is greatest. In London in 2012 there were 32,000 people living with HIV who were diagnosed and having treatment and an estimated further 6,000-plus who were undiagnosed. Eighteen of the twenty local authorities with the highest HIV prevalence were in London. The worst placed was Lambeth with a prevalence of 1.4 per cent. As with Washington DC, the comparison should not be exaggerated, but such a prevalence is on a par with some sub-Saharan African countries. Yet Lambeth is just over the river from the Houses of Parliament and in easy sight from the windows of both the House of Commons and the House of Lords. Just as in the United States, it seems that the biggest problem is in the shadow of the very seat of national government.

Of course it is true that if you take the British figures as a whole they are not on the scale of sub-Saharan Africa – and the same applies to the vast majority of West European countries. We might remember, however, that if you put all the countries of Western and Central Europe together, UNAIDS estimates that there are now approaching a million people living with HIV. In France there are probably about 150,000; in Italy around 125,000; and in Spain between 140,000 at the lower estimate and 170,000 at the higher. As for prevalence the UNAIDS estimates show Germany at 0.2 per cent; United Kingdom at 0.3 per cent and France at 0.4 per cent. Only Estonia and Latvia break the 1 per cent measure – although Portugal comes close. If you were to ask for one common problem it would be the fifth to a quarter who are undiagnosed, and if you ask for a common solution it would be more testing.

But is more testing the only way forward? Surely if you provided antiretroviral drugs right from the beginning when a man or woman is most infectious, that would cut the onward transmission rate dramatically. In other words, give antiretrovirals as soon as the man or woman is infected rather than wait until their CD4 count reaches some WHO threshold. In 2013 the incomparable Health Protection Agency produced a report on a five-year study of men who have sex with men. It went to the heart of the central issue in this book. How do you reduce the infectivity of this group? Can transmission of HIV be controlled by universal access to antiretroviral drugs?

The agency (now part of Health Protection England) found that about a quarter of men having sex with men were undiagnosed and many others who may have been diagnosed, for one reason or another, were not adhering to their treatment. Self-evidently, these two groups would be largely unaffected by a policy of antiretroviral drugs for everyone and this substantially reduces the potential for the success of any policy of extending treatment. If, on the other hand, the policy was combined with improving the numbers of the tested and ensuring more frequent testing and adherence then that would substantially reduce the number of undiagnosed. Interestingly, Dr Andrew Phillips of University College London came to almost exactly the same conclusion using a mathematical model. His research, based on the figures of men having sex with men, showed that, by itself, the extension of drug provision would have limited effect. However, if you increased testing and also provided immediate and universal antiretroviral treatment then you could achieve a dramatic fall in HIV transmission.

Some will say that it is a big 'if' to assume that substantially increased testing can be achieved – and so it is on the basis of past experience. But perhaps all that proves is that past campaigns have been low profile and frankly lacklustre. I do not remember a campaign in London on the Washington model of 'Come together DC – Get Screened for HIV'. I cannot remember posters setting out such a message. I cannot recall when the health service was last given the budget to attempt such an obvious step forward. I wonder just how many in London actually know anything about the undiagnosed let alone the importance of people living with HIV sticking to their treatment.

In the absence of a vaccine my own view is that a further extension of antiretroviral treatment holds out the best hope of making a dramatic reduction in new infections. In the next chapter I set out the policies that I believe would help further. For Britain I stress two. The need to lift the generally abysmal level of sex education in schools; and the need for government to support the excellent research which will never be taken on by the commercial pharmaceutical companies. There is one further point that needs to be underlined. The National Health Service has come in for more than its fair share of criticism in the last few years. Yet, in the case of public health it is one of the reasons why Britain has a relatively high proportion of people living with HIV who have an undetectable viral load and who, other things being equal, will not pass on the infection. As Professor Anderson says,

> *The National Health Service works on the basis of clinical need, not an individual's ability to pay, which means that HIV diagnosis and treatment is freely available for everyone who needs them. For HIV, associated as it is with poverty and marginalisation, it's a principle that must be uncompromisingly upheld.*

In several other respects the British contribution has been substantial. In 2014 Action for Global Health, an organisation of fifteen non-government organisations and charities based in Europe, examined the contribution that six European Union countries – France, Germany, Italy, the Netherlands, Spain and Britain – make to the health systems of overseas countries. Generally it found that 'most European governments are either decreasing their overseas development assistance for health as a percentage of gross national income or their contributions are stagnating at low levels'. Britain was the only country to have steadily increased its health contribution.

At home a massive step forward was taken to reduce the prejudice against gay people by introducing the 2013 equal marriage legislation. For the Prime Minister, David Cameron, it held no party advantage – as the resignations from local Conservative associations showed – but the big majorities in the House of Commons and House of Lords must surely have given encouragement to those who were prevented by fear and stigma of accessing medical treatment. Another important measure was the decision to give free HIV treatment to political asylum applicants straight away rather than after a six-month wait – which was a policy that had made no sense and simply allowed HIV to spread. Of course, not all the advances have come from the government or the health service. Britain has been immeasurably helped by a whole series of civil society organisations, ranging from service providers like the Terrence Higgins Trust to the skilled campaigners of the National Aids Trust, to the multitude of big and small organisations outside government that are too numerous to mention. Some have been working since the 1980s, often against a background of stretched financial resources, and without their contribution we would not have managed.

All told Britain has a decent record – which makes it all the stranger to come across palpably bad decisions like the cuts to the funding of vaccine research, and by an odd reluctance to proclaim what the government is doing. There was no minister at the World Aids Conference in 2012 to set out British policy, and the government shows acute nervousness about announcing policies that could offend those who oppose giving overseas aid. Even more extraordinarily, the doubling of the contribution to the Global Fund in late 2013 was barely publicised domestically. At the health department, I saw for myself the nervousness with which preparations were made to accept what happened to be my amendment in the House of Lords for extending HIV treatment for asylum seekers. The spin doctors went to work; the pitch was rolled; the public should be prepared. The result was a pre-announcement in the *Daily Telegraph* with the splash headline 'Foreigners to be Offered Free Treatment for HIV on the NHS'.

Perhaps the nervousness results from the criticism aimed at David Cameron in the wake of the marriage equality bill. If so I think it is profoundly mistaken. The spin doctors will always advise caution on money going to what they perceive as unpopular causes. My view would be that the only chance you have of winning this argument is to take it full on and come out fighting.

A more fundamental question which waits to be decided is the outcome of the government's decision on the organisation of public health. It decided to ring-fence the public health budget which (provided the budget is adequate) is a sensible change. More contentious is the decision to hand over responsibility for public health to local councils. Supporters of the change say that local councils are in the best position to make decisions on the public health needs of their own areas. It seems based on the premise that the National Health Service is not capable of being local, which in my experience is nonsense. The concern is that HIV expertise is firmly inside the health service and the fear is that some councils will not give the priority to HIV, drugs and sex work that the health service has done over the years. It also runs the risk of being a recipe for confusion and a disjointed, patchy approach. There are thirty councils in London alone, and funding is provided against a backdrop of shrinking resources for local government. It is a policy that needs to be kept under close review and it would help also if there was some consistency in Whitehall itself; since 2000 there have been no fewer than nine public health ministers.

My (doubtless naïve) ambition in 1986 was to make Britain an example of what could be achieved in tackling HIV and Aids. Under different governments, we have made undoubted progress. Back in the 1980s almost everyone with HIV died; today in Britain almost everyone with HIV infection lives. The position has been transformed but we must not give up now. Our problems are obviously less than sub-Saharan Africa or Eastern Europe, but that gives us an opportunity to show what can be done. We should see how more people with HIV can be persuaded into treatment, how HIV can be further prevented and how treatment can be extended and improved. We should face down the discrimination and prejudice there is against sexual minorities as well as against drug users and sex workers. So it seems to me that the answer to my question in the title of this chapter is that, self-evidently, HIV – and all the issues around it – continues to be a problem in Britain. We have made undoubted progress since the 1980s, but there is a long way to go. HIV may have slipped out of the headlines, but we should avoid any false assurances that the battle is almost won or HIV is no longer a problem. Any politician or minister at Westminster who attempts to claim that it is should be unceremoniously dumped in the Thames and told to swim over to Lambeth.

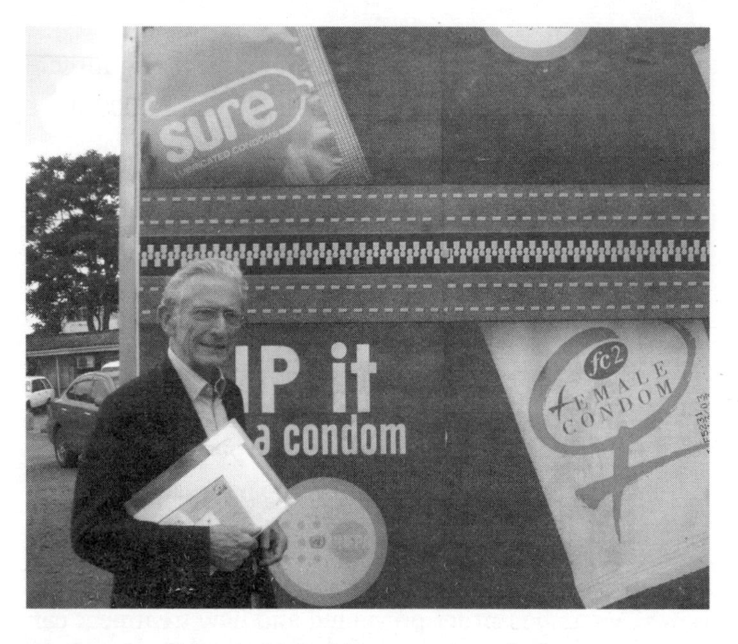

Direct advertising in Nairobi – an approach that many countries in the West now ignore.

ELEVEN

WHAT DO WE DO NEXT?

THE CENTRAL PROBLEM that the world faces with HIV and Aids today is this: it is the millions of people infected with HIV who, in spite of the medical advances and all the money poured in to help, remain untreated. The solution involves immensely more than the provision of extra antiretroviral drugs. UNAIDS estimate that about half of people living with HIV are also undiagnosed. That means that around eighteen million people in the world today are living in ignorance of their condition. *Eighteen million.* The danger is twofold. There is the obvious danger to those who are infected, but there is the additional danger to public health generally. People with untreated HIV can spread the virus further. It means that hospitals and clinics are involved in a perpetual struggle to catch up. For every person they put on treatment there are approaching two others somewhere in the world acquiring HIV for the first time. How on earth can you defeat Aids against that background? We need policies that meet the needs of those who are waiting for treatment but at the same time reduce the colossal number of the undiagnosed. No one should be under any illusion about the barriers that stand in the way.

We need first to radically reduce the number of the undiagnosed living in ignorance of their condition. The longer treatment is delayed the more difficult it is. Even those who reach treatment may find their life expectancy curtailed. And of course not knowing of their condition they can easily pass on the virus. Not everyone does but, as we have seen in London, a fifth of those with HIV are undiagnosed but that fifth is responsible for over half of new infections. London is one city which, by international standards, has a relatively low number of people living with HIV; in many other cities the numbers involved will be immense.

Then there are those who know they have HIV and who have begun treatment, but for one reason or another do not continue. The danger, as we saw in Washington, is that once they slip out of treatment their HIV becomes harder to treat when and if they eventually return, and in the meantime they become infectious again. This issue is given little publicity. The public assumption is that if treatment is given it will be accepted and automatically followed. Self-evidently that is not the case.

Lastly there are the men and women who have HIV and are waiting in a queue for treatment. The latest WHO guidance from Geneva brings forward the time when treatment should be started, but even those guidelines exclude most of the very newly infected. These people may be in no imminent danger themselves, but they are at their most infectious at this stage and pose the greatest danger to others.

The medical goal for people living with HIV is to achieve an undetectable viral load, which means that, to all intents and purposes, they cannot pass on the virus to others. The figures show just how far we are away from reaching that aim. In the United States less than a third of men and women living with HIV reach that goal. Across the Atlantic in Britain and France almost 60 per cent reach the goal, but that still leaves 40 per cent who do not. If this is the position in the rich West what is it in countries that do not have such wealth, where public health systems are undeveloped, and where travel difficulties are all too real?

It is difficult to see how, without further action around the world, HIV and Aids can be defeated. That is not a criticism of the dedicated work of clinicians, international and civil society organisations and volunteers. It is a recognition that they need more help and that they need it urgently if even more lives are not going to be squandered. That help must come from governments, for that is where responsibility lies. The need is for a renewed international effort. I would propose ten measures which would help avert at least part of the continuing tragedy:

First, there must be a new initiative on prevention. As a world we seem much more prepared to pay for the casualties of HIV than to prevent them. There are no demonstrations outside the White House in Washington, or the Parliament building in Cape Town, or down Whitehall in London, calling for more prevention. There have been plenty calling for more treatment. Although it is entirely right that those who already have HIV should insist on treatment, it is also right that the public should insist that every effort is made to stop the disease spreading. With over thirty-five million living with HIV and another thirty-six million already dead, our progress is painfully and tragically slow. One reason is that the resources devoted to prevention do not bear any comparison with the money devoted to treatment.

Let me give an example from Britain, which is obviously the country I know best. When I chaired the all-party House of Lords Select Committee on HIV which reported on the position in September 2011, we pointed out that although the nation spent approaching £1 billion a year on antiretroviral treatment and care, the Department of Health spent only £4.9 million a year on health promotion and advertising to prevent HIV. I found the prevention figure so incomprehensibly low that I asked for it to be checked three times. When we found it was accurate, the committee urged an increase. The response from the health department was to cut the amount to £4.45 million. It must rate as one of the most short-sighted policies ever, but the trouble is that it is exactly the kind of priority that is being given to health promotion around the globe.

We need to recognise that determined efforts on publicity in the past have not failed, but have been successful. Both in Britain and Australia the big advertising campaigns (although controversial with some) reduced the numbers contracting HIV as well as other sexually transmitted diseases. But, like all other campaigns, they needed to develop and be consistently put to the public. Coca-Cola would not mount a major campaign one year and then go off the air for the next quarter of a century. We need to use all the means open to us which were not available back in the 1980s, like the internet and social media, while not ignoring the more traditional means of communication. Over the years in New York and Washington I have seen posters and advertisements on the subways. In Kenya I saw the poster vans. I cannot remember a similar effort in Moscow – or, for that matter, in most cities in Western Europe. In short we need to return to public education and use some of the messages from the past. Risky behaviour still needs to be changed, the numbers of partners need to be reduced and condoms still need to be used.

Second, the highest priority in public education should go to increasing testing. If we can bring the number of the undiagnosed down then we will have taken a major step to reducing HIV – assuming that testing is followed by treatment. The aim must be to ensure that tests are provided in the places that are most convenient to the public and that results do not leak into an intolerant community. That is why home testing is so important. Testing takes place conveniently and privately with the offer of swift confirmation of the results and counselling. In every nation there are testing opportunities – like the tests offered to the drivers in Washington DC waiting for their licenses to be renewed, or patients in the waiting rooms of surgeries, or prisoners entering prison. HIV is no longer a death sentence but a long-term condition. A positive diagnosis can still be traumatic but is not the utterly shattering event of twenty-five years ago. The aim must be to make HIV tests a normal part of medical checks.

Third, sensible sex and relationship education should be introduced. In some parts of the world there is vast ignorance. In Yangon (previously Rangoon) I was told by one of the few campaigners there that the issue was that young people and many others still ask 'What is HIV?' In the West ignorance is not usually on that scale (although it can be), but everyone will tell you that the level of knowledge is nothing like what it was at the end of the 1980s. There is ignorance about how HIV is transmitted and there is ignorance about the precautions to be taken. In many countries efforts to change the position are defeated by the churches. The arguments used remain very much the kind of reservations that Margaret Thatcher had and which are described in my first chapter: that education will expose children to new knowledge that will be damaging and should be postponed until much later. The difficulty is that the 'much later' never comes. The assumption that parents carry out this part of education is highly optimistic. As I have travelled around the world I have been struck by the large numbers of parents, as well as clinicians, who instead favour action in schools.

Fourth, antiretroviral treatment should be offered to *all* people with HIV as soon after they are infected as possible. Up until very recently we have been giving treatment only when the patient enters the danger zone. This was defined by the WHO as when the CD4 count in the blood fell below 350 micro litres of blood. They have now adjusted that lower limit to a CD4 count of below 500. It is a major step forward, although I accept that some countries still cannot reach the old limit. But to my mind there seems no reason why there should be a limit of any kind. All clinicians agree that HIV is dramatically more infectious just after it has been contracted. Surely it makes no sense to exclude the most infectious from drug treatment.

The almost automatic reaction of governments is to shudder at the cost. But there is another way of looking at the position. If your aim is to reduce the amount of onward transmission, then clearly the greater the number on treatment and adhering to it the better. Other things being equal, prevention reduces the number with HIV and saves the onward and permanent cost of treatment. The greater access to generics over the next few years gives governments the cost opportunity to introduce this policy. Governments might remember that sooner or later they are going to have to put people with HIV on treatment in any event.

There has already been encouraging evidence about what can be achieved by extending treatment to anyone with HIV, regardless of their blood count, and more could be provided by pilot schemes. As for the argument that people given such treatment will need to adhere to it, that is an argument that already applies to the existing situation. Whatever happens, campaigns on improving adherence will be necessary and we will need more testing if such a change in policy is to stand any chance of success. There are obvious difficulties for countries which even now cannot reach everyone below the WHO limit, but for others there is the chance of getting off the escalator of ever-rising numbers of people with HIV.

Fifth, the ultimate goal is to develop a vaccine. The polio vaccine has eradicated that condition in my lifetime. After the war I remember the children who were crippled with polio, the warnings not to use public swimming pools and the pictures in magazines of the unhappy prisoners in their iron lungs. That has now been eradicated in virtually every nation of the world, the only exceptions being where there are religious and political objections to vaccination itself. An Aids vaccine could have an equally dramatic effect and mean that the vast cost of treatment would be progressively reduced. You would think that hardly anything could be more important, but the truth is that the search for an Aids vaccine has been under-resourced. More resources would speed up the process and mean that new avenues could be explored. The pharmaceutical industry shows little inclination to invest: the risk is too high and the likely financial reward too low. This means that any advance for the benefit of the public is down to governments and foundations. The United States shoulders the bulk of the burden, although in all conscience there is no reason why they should be so unsupported by other nations. It is time that all the rich countries of the world stepped up to the plate. They should remember the words of Peter Piot, speaking in 2014, who said, 'Ending HIV without a vaccine will simply not be possible.' My case rests.

Sixth, we must tackle in a much more determined way the corruption which scars so many nations today. It has been a constant complaint on my travels. Police taking pay-offs, officials creaming off government funds, politicians taking bribes. The lowest form of corruption is when it deprives patients of medicines and drugs which can save their lives. The successors to Harry Lime in Graham Greene's *The Third Man* are alive today and thriving.

Corruption also has another effect. The fact that there is corruption at all deters governments from giving to overseas aid programmes (including aid to improve health systems) and provides a useful stick for the opponents of such aid. Even a squeaky-clean and open organisation like the Global Fund in Geneva gets tarnished by the generalised charges. Where possible, money should be directed straight to civil society organisations working on the ground, or through agencies like the Global Fund. The standards of the civil society organisations I have seen are high, as too is the motivation of those who work for them – often in the most difficult of conditions.

Seventh, if we are to tackle corruption then we must tackle the question of sex work, which also has a major impact on HIV. Around the world sex workers are exploited. They are exploited by their pimps, by their landlords and by the police. They are treated as outcasts and forced to work in the shadows. Health care is neglected and the inevitable result is that in all too many nations the prevalence of HIV infection among sex workers is way above that of the general population. Frequently, what makes this possible are the hypocritical and counter-productive laws that cover the area and which mean that around the globe sex work is overwhelmingly marked down as criminal. In reality it is widely tolerated, provided that as much as possible it is kept out of sight, and the usual official defence is that even though it is technically illegal the law is 'lightly' enforced. The trouble with this argument is that the lack of certainty gives the green light to corrupt policemen and anyone else who wants to take advantage of the position. New South Wales is one of the few exceptions to the general rule. In Sydney sex work is run under normal business controls and as a result there has been no recent case of HIV being passed on by a sex worker and police corruption in this area has been virtually eliminated. A debate has now started on the position in other countries. In Western Europe an argument that has gained ground is that only the client should be penalised – and that a determined new policy of this kind would much better protect the sex worker. The counter-argument to that is that this will still push much sex work outside the law and will certainly require a police effort to enforce what will be a new criminal offence. Nevertheless, it is a debate which needs to be joined if we are ever to make any progress. We might remember that in Sydney the changes to the state law followed the exposure by official investigations of the deeply unsatisfactory position that existed while sex work remained illegal. Other cities would also benefit from such investigations, including not only New Delhi and Kiev, but also London.

Eighth, the success of the harm-reduction policies in drugs policy must be shouted loud. The provision of clean needles and syringes has been an undoubted success. As we have seen, where such policies are implemented, new infections from HIV by shared needles have been reduced to remarkably low figures and, in spite of some of the fears, neither crime nor drug taking has risen as a result. In Britain it is also an interesting supporting argument for those who think that drugs policy should be put under the charge of the Health Department and not the Home Office. Nothing I or anyone else says is likely to persuade Russia from its woeful and deadly path in refusing to countenance such a policy, but the United States is different. There, many states have their own clean-needle policies. Their success has been established. The message to Congress is to please look at the evidence again and then end the ban on federal funds being used for such schemes. Such a decision would not only bring in much needed resources, but would send a message around the world. At the same time all nations should note the initiative of the United Nations General Secretary, Ban Ki-moon, in calling a special session of the General Assembly on illicit drugs in September 2016. This initiative gives a perfect focus for the discussions that are already going on in so many countries and offers an opportunity for the introduction of new policies that more surely penalise the traffickers and not the users.

Ninth, a new dialogue must be attempted with the churches and the faith leaders. They have the power to change attitudes, but it has been one of the most depressing features of my travels to find so many churches arm in arm with the most reactionary political elements in the world. Goodness knows there are many religions but I would have thought that all were united in offering help to the disadvantaged – like the minorities who feature so prominently in the HIV area. Yet, we have the Orthodox churches in Russia and Ukraine that fail to challenge public intolerance on homosexuality. We have the Roman Catholic Church clinging to a policy of banning condom use, which has been responsible for a multitude of deaths from Aids and goes smack against any concept of a right to life. And then, perhaps worst of all for me personally, we find the Anglican Church in Africa, and particularly Uganda, supporting some of the most discriminatory laws in the world. As a church, the Anglicans seem to have a particular difficulty with homosexuality, and even in Britain you find the bishops deciding that the civil right of equal marriage should not be available to their own clergy. They should beware, lest their reputation for intolerance spread.

Tenth, politicians must start leading again. Enormous progress was made, particularly in the first years of the twenty-first century, thanks to the efforts of politicians, clinicians and activists of every conceivable hue working together. In 2003 we had a Republican President of the richest country on earth prepared to commit his nation to supporting the permanent medical treatment of millions of men and women, thousands of miles from his political base. For George W. Bush, there was almost no political advantage in establishing PEPFAR, but he did it all the same because it was right. In 2002 we had nations coming together to set up the Global Fund which would funnel resources to where they were most needed. The funds were not labelled by nation, but were given freely to be distributed according to need and without thought of commercial or national return. These were actions of principle. They recognised the duty that the comparatively rich have to the grindingly poor.

The commitment of the clinicians, the civil society organisations and the volunteers remains, but the commitment of the politicians is at worst absent and at best wavering. Politicians in countries like Russia and Uganda are content to preside over death and discrimination. Politicians in countries like Ukraine (certainly up to now) have done the very least they can get away with. And too many politicians in the United States and Britain either back their own prejudices or are nervous of being seen to espouse the cause of minorities who they believe are unpopular with the public and, of course, the brutish section of the media.

We should remember that most major failures have come about because of a lack of political leadership, a lack of political courage, or a refusal to look at the facts. As we have seen, in South Africa the issue was practically ignored by one leader and then steered on a ridiculously damaging course by his successor. But what South Africa also demonstrated was that when new politicians took over with new policies that were guided by evidence and not by unsubstantiated belief, then the results could be remarkably positive. It is an example to politicians in all nations of what can be achieved.

The world now stands at a tipping point. We can go forward and develop new policies that give us some hope of defeating HIV and Aids, or we can sink into a sea of complacence, wrongly believing it was all yesterday's problem. If we go forward then we must overcome one last barrier which still stands in our way: the barrier of prejudice, which can defeat all our efforts.

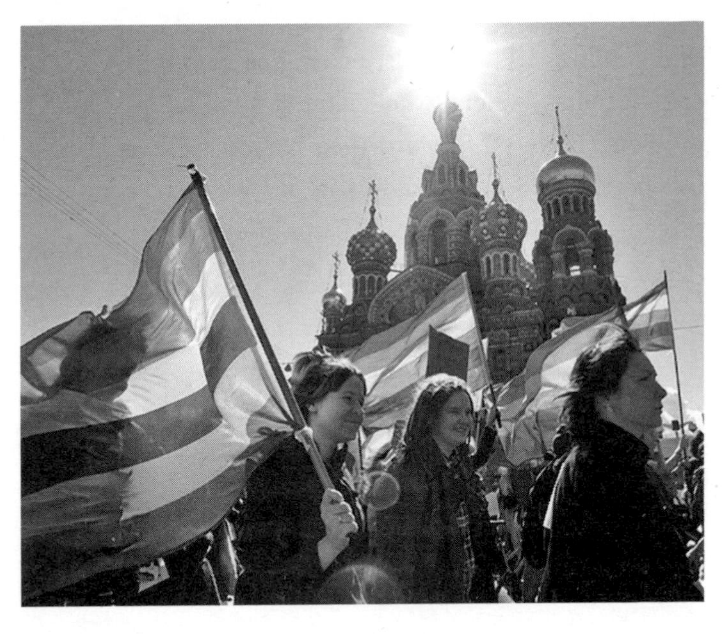

Fighting injustice – a gay rights demonstration in 2013 in St Petersburg.

TWELVE

ENDPIECE: THE SHAME OF THE WORLD

WHEN THE PRESIDENT of Uganda finally signed the new repressive laws aimed directly at gay people, the country turned its back on decency and human rights. That much is clear. The World Bank suspended new loans for the health service and Denmark, Norway and the Netherlands halted aid. But the point which was so often ignored in the aftermath was that around the world there are many Ugandas. What has shocked me most in my travels has been the degree of prejudice which I have found. Of course I knew it existed but to my discredit I had never realised the depth of it. I had not realised that drug users would be left to die in Russia or that the Americans would support their callous policies. I had not realised that sex workers would be so gravely exploited in India or suffer so many murders in Britain. And I certainly had not realised the depth of feeling that exists against gay men, lesbian women and transgender people around the world, leading to some of the worst persecution that has taken place since the end of the Second World War.

Today, same-sex relations are criminal in the majority of African countries. The only feature which sets Uganda apart is the severity of the repression – although even in that they are run close by Nigeria. But the prejudice is not remotely confined to Africa. In almost eighty countries of the world homosexuality remains a criminal offence, including in India, the largest democracy in the world. In Russia new laws have been passed to counter an invented threat to children but which the opinion polls show are supported by the public. In other countries gay men are imprisoned and in Iran they have been hanged. Even when the law has been changed it has not always transformed attitudes. In Ukraine and much of Eastern Europe the hostility persists, to the extent that the hero of the Polish uprising, Lech Walesa, said in March 2013 that gays had no right to sit on the front benches in Parliament and should sit at the back – 'even behind a wall'.

In West Europe the prejudice is usually not so extreme but in its own way it is just as pernicious. London is meant to be the gay capital of Europe, but a gay friend of mine told me that if he went down any street in Britain hand-in-hand with his long-term partner he would be met by abuse and possibly worse. The House of Bishops in the Church of England have banned their own clergy from entering into same-sex marriage, even though it is now the law of the land. Or take the football terraces. One footballer complained that he was barracked because a part of the crowd thought wrongly that he was gay. If he had been we assume that the abuse would have been even more heartfelt and it certainly explains why virtually no professional footballer has come out.

From the point of view of this book this prejudice has a disastrous impact upon the fight against HIV. Where there are criminal laws against homosexuality, gay people are not going to come forward for testing and treatment if they believe they risk prosecution. If they do come forward it may be at a very late stage of the disease when treatment is most difficult and when their life expectancy has been reduced – if not snuffed out. The reason is quite clear. They fear that news about their sexual orientation will leak into the local community and make their own position untenable. Time and time again in different countries I have been told how young men have been forced out of their family homes in the face of community hostility.

And of course it is not only gay people who suffer. I remember too well the transgender people in India hoping against hope for acceptance. I remember also the discrimination against people who have contracted HIV. So often the woman is blamed even when she has been infected by her husband or partner. Women living with HIV fear that knowledge of their illness will doom them to a life of isolation; men fear they will be shunned at work or lose their jobs altogether. In 2012 I went to Skopje, the capital of Macedonia (one of the smallest countries in the world), to encourage the formation of a parliamentary group like the one at Westminster. After a series of media interviews our small party made our way to dinner past the outsize statue of Alexander the Great. As we walked I said to one of the local organisers that he must appear regularly on radio and television. He had been diagnosed with HIV eighteen months previously. 'No,' he replied, 'I am not that brave.'

The position with HIV points to a much wider issue. The basic human rights of millions of men and women around the world are now under sustained attack. Surely people of good will must combat this in a much more powerful way than we have managed up to now. So how can we begin to change the prejudice and the discrimination? I made some proposals in the last chapter and some of the opportunities are available immediately. India has the opportunity of scrapping at long last the 150-year-old laws which criminalise homosexuality and were made by the British colonial government in a different age. Australia has the opportunity of passing a federal law to allow equal marriage which not only would do good for many gay couples but would also burnish their reputation for sensible policy making. And the United States should lift the federal ban on clean-needle schemes which would not only do good but also save lives. Each one of those actions requires the decision of politicians and, if taken, would send a message around the world. Above all, they would be a check on the wave of repression which is currently sweeping too much before it.

Disgracefully, the position of the minorities that I write about in this book has, if anything, become worse over the last eighteen months. If I was a gay man living in many countries today I would compare my position to that of being black and living under apartheid in South Africa, or being a Jew living under the Nazis in Germany. That really is the shame of the world. It is time for those of us who believe that this is an international scandal on a par with race and religious hatred to combat the bigots and to find a way forward. An international convention to protect their rights would self-evidently not win the approval of all nations but many would support it. An international conference in London could explore this and other options. The importance of London as a venue would be to demonstrate once and for all that the world has moved on. It is no longer a defence to say that many of the laws against homosexuality were introduced by Britain. That was in the nineteenth century, and today we have new and better values. Our aim in the twenty-first century should be to support people who by any standard are oppressed and to encourage those who are discriminated against to claim their rights. If we could achieve this it would also be, in the terms of this book, an enormous step forward in defeating HIV and Aids.

APPENDIX

DON'T DIE OF IGNORANCE

AIDS

DON'T DIE OF IGNORANCE

GOVERNMENT INFORMATION 1987

WHY ARE YOU BEING SENT THIS LEAFLET ? 1

This leaflet is being sent to every household in the country. It is about AIDS. And everyone now needs to know the facts. It explains what the disease is. How it is spread. How serious a threat it is. And how it can be avoided.

Because it has to deal with matters of health and sex, you may find some of the information disturbing. But please make sure that everyone who may need this advice reads this leaflet.

The more people know about AIDS, the less likely it is to be spread.

So if you have children, think carefully what they need to know. Whether you approve or not, many teenagers do have sex and some may experiment with drugs.

Even if you think your children don't, they will need advice because they may have friends who encourage them to.

WHY SHOULD YOU BE CONCERNED ABOUT AIDS ? 2

Any man or woman can get the AIDS virus depending on their behaviour. It is not just a homosexual disease.

There is no cure. And it kills.

By the time you read this, probably 300 people will have died in this country. It is believed that a further 30,000 carry the virus. This number is rising and will continue to rise unless we all take precautions.

WHAT IS AIDS ? 3

AIDS is caused by a virus. This can attack the body's defence system which normally helps fight off diseases and infections.

And if this happens people can then develop AIDS – the disease itself. They become ill and die from illnesses they cannot fight off.

HOW DO YOU BECOME INFECTED ? 4

Because the virus can be present in semen and vaginal fluid, this means for most people the only real danger comes through having sexual intercourse with an infected person. This means vaginal or anal sex. (It could also be that oral sex can be risky particularly if semen is taken into the mouth.)

So the virus can be passed from man to man, man to woman and woman to man.

For those who inject drugs, there is the added risk from sharing needles or equipment with someone who is infected.

Finally, babies born to mothers who are infected have a high chance of being born with the virus.

HOW CAN YOU PROTECT YOURSELF FROM AIDS ? 5

Most people who have the virus don't even know it. They may look and feel completely well. So you cannot know who is infected and who isn't. To protect yourself follow these guidelines.

The more sexual partners you have, especially male partners, the more chance you have of having sex with someone who is infected. It is safest to stick to one faithful partner.

FEWER PARTNERS, LESS RISK.

Unless you are sure of your partner, always use a condom (sheath or rubber). This will reduce the risk of catching the virus.

USE CONDOMS FOR SAFER SEX.

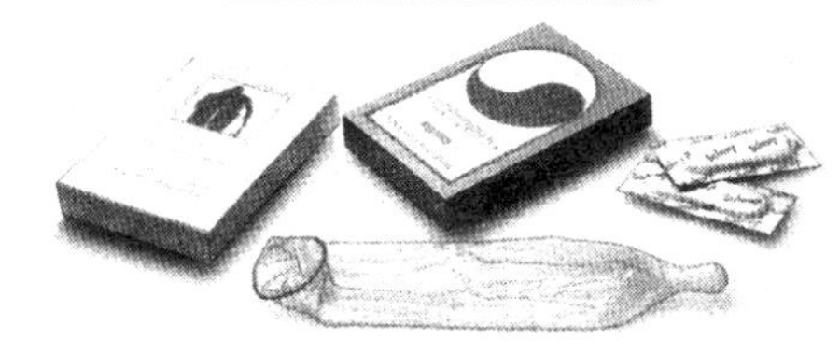

It's also best to use a water-based lubricating gel with the condom. Oil-based gels can weaken the rubber. Ask your chemist for advice.

The contraceptive pill is no protection against AIDS.

Anyone who misuses drugs should not inject. If you ever do, never share equipment (needles, syringes, mixing bowls, etc.). You could be injecting the virus straight into your blood stream. It is extremely dangerous.

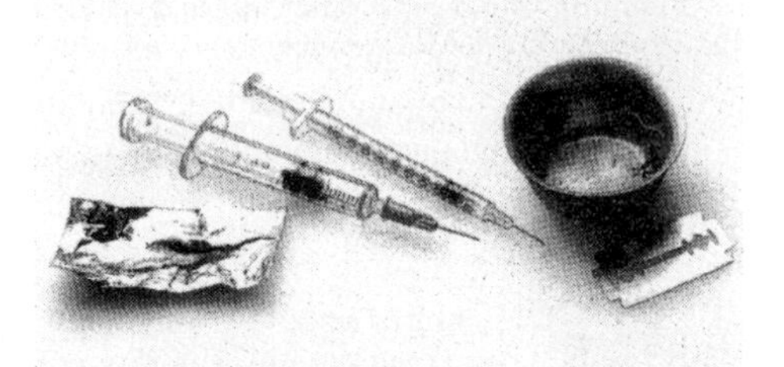

DON'T INJECT. NEVER SHARE.

IF YOU THINK YOU ARE INFECTED ? 6

If you think you may be infected go to your family doctor for advice about having a test. Or go direct to a clinic for sexually transmitted diseases for confidential advice and a test if you wish. If you have the virus, they'll let you know and give you help and support.

WHAT ABOUT THINGS THAT PIERCE THE SKIN ? 7

It is *not* safe to use equipment for ear-piercing, tattooing or acupuncture unless you know it is unused or has been sterilised. Nor is it safe to share a toothbrush or razor of someone who is infected. These things could give you the virus through infected blood.

WHAT CAN'T YOU CATCH THE VIRUS FROM ?

8

The Government's clear medical advice is that you cannot get the AIDS virus from normal social contact with someone who is infected.

You cannot get it from shaking hands. Nor is there any record of anyone becoming infected through kissing.

There is no danger in sharing cups or cutlery. Nor can you catch it from public baths or toilets.

In hospitals, standard disinfection precautions protect patients, visitors and staff.

Giving blood is safe. All the equipment is only used once.

And all the blood used in this country for blood transfusion is rigorously checked.

HOW SAFE IS IT ABROAD ?

9

The AIDS virus exists throughout the world. In certain areas a large number of both men and women have it.

So it is even more important that you follow the advice in this leaflet if you're going abroad.

Otherwise if you do have sex with someone who is not your usual partner, not only might you become infected, but you may also infect your partner when you return home.

Again, in some countries blood transfusions are not checked for the AIDS virus. In those places where the virus is widespread do not, if you can possibly avoid it, have blood from a local donor.

Also, in certain developing countries, medical equipment may not be properly sterilised. If you can, avoid any treatment involving injections and surgical procedures.

If you have any worries about this, discuss them with your family doctor.

DO YOU NEED MORE INFORMATION ?

10

The true picture about AIDS is that, at the moment, relatively few have the virus in this country. Those most at risk now are men who have anal sex with other men. Drug misusers who share equipment. Anyone with many sexual partners. And sexual partners of any of these people.

But the virus *is* spreading. And as it does, so the risk of having sex with someone who is infected increases.

Ultimately, defence against the disease depends on all of us taking responsibility for our own actions.

More detailed information is available from:
Your own doctor.
Clinics for sexually transmitted diseases. (Look in the phone book under Venereal or Sexually Transmitted Diseases or your nearest main hospital.)
Healthline Telephone Service 01-981 2717, 01-980 7222, 0345-581151. (If you're phoning from outside London, use the 0345 number and you'll be charged at local rates.)
Terrence Higgins Trust 01-833 2971.
Welsh AIDS Campaign 0222-464121.
Scottish AIDS Monitor 031-558 1167.
London Lesbian and Gay Switchboard 01-837 7324.
SCODA (Standing Conference on Drug Abuse) 01-430 2341.

For a copy of the more detailed booklet AIDS: What Everybody Needs to Know, write to Dept. A, PO Box 100, Milton Keynes, MK1 1TX. (In Scotland write for The AIDS Problem: What Everybody Needs to Know, to the Scottish Health Education Group, Woodburn House, Canaan Lane, Edinburgh EH10 4SG.)

If you're travelling abroad, read leaflet SA35, Protect Your Health Abroad, available from travel agents.

D O N'T A I D A I D S

Issued by the Department of Health and Social Security.
Printed in the U.K. for HMSO. 1986. Dd 8934260 HSSHJ0258.

BIBLIOGRAPHY

For this book I found a number of reports and books particularly useful. First and foremost there are the annual Global Reports of UNAIDS, together with a series of other reports they publish . Both the WHO and the Global Fund also publish their own reports and most other countries publish figures on their latest positions. For example, in London there are reports from the Health Protection Agency; in the United States from the Centre for Disease Control; in India there is the National AIDS Control Organisation; and in Australia there is the Kirby Institute.

Among the books I would recommend are:

- William Dalrymple, *City of Djinns: A Year in Delhi,* (London: Flamingo, 1999)
- Peter Piot, *No Time to Lose,* 1st ed. (London: W.W. Norton and Company, 2012)
- Anna Reid, *Borderland: A Journey through the History of Ukraine*, (London: Basic Books, 2000)
- Craig Timberg and Daniel Halperin, *Tinderbox: How the West Sparked the AIDS Epidemic and How the World Can Finally Overcome it*, 1st ed. (London: Penguin Books, 2012)

The reports I draw from for this book include:

- *The War on Drugs and HIV/AIDS: How the Criminalisation of the Drug Use Fuels the Global Pandemic,* Global Commission on Drug Policy, June 2012.
- *Who Pays for Health? Trends in Official Development Assistance for Health,* Action for Global Health, December 2013.
- *Time to Test for HIV: Expanded Healthcare and Community HIV Testing in England,* Health Protection Agency, December 2010.

- *HIV: Public Knowledge and Attitudes*, National AIDS Trust, January 2011.
- *HIV Prevention Needs Assessment for London,* Future Commissioning of London HIV Prevention Services Project Steering Group, Association of Directors of Public Health, Public Health England, London Councils, 2013.
- *No Vaccine, No Cure: HIV and AIDS in the United Kingdom,* Select Committee on HIV and AIDS in the United Kingdom, 1st Report of Session 2010-12, 2011.
- Brown, A.E., Gill, O.N. and Delpech V.C. 'HIV Treatment as prevention among men who have sex with men in the UK: is transmission controlled by universal access to HIV treatment and care? *HIV Medicine* (2013), 9, pp. 563-570.
- *HIV Infection in Scotland. Report of the Scottish Committee on HIV Infection and Intravenous Drug Use.* Scottish Office Home and Health Department Edinburgh, Scottish Office, 1986.
- *The Wolfenden Report on Homosexual Offences and Prostitution*, London: HMSO, September 4, 1957.
- *Financing the Response to HIV in Low- and Middle-Income Countries: International Assistance from Donor Governments in 2012*, The Henry J. Kaiser Family Foundation, September 2013.
- *Prevention and Treatment of HIV and Other Sexually Transmitted Infections among Men who have Sex with Men and Transgender People: Recommendations for a Public Health Approach,* World Health Organisation, 2011.
- *Prevention and Treatment of HIV and Other Sexually Transmitted Infections for Sex Workers in Low- and Middle- Income Countries: Recommendations for a Public Health Approach,* World Health Organisation, December 2012.
- *The Strategic Use of Antiretrovirals to Help End the HIV Epidemic,* World Health Organisation, 2012.
- *"Atmospheric Pressure": Russian Drug Policy as a Driver for Violations of the UN Convention Against Torture*, Andrey Rylkov Foundation, Canadian HIV/AIDS Legal Network, Eurasian Harm Reduction Network, 2011.
- Nebrenchina, Luba *Drug Policy in Russia: Drug Users' Stories of Repression*, (Moscow: The Andrey Rylkov Foundation for Health and Social Justice, 2009).
- Bobrova, Natalia et al. 'Challenges in providing drug user treatment services in Russia: providers' views' *Substance Use & Misuse* (2008), 43, pp. 1770-1784.
- Latypov, Alisher B. 'The Soviet Doctor and the treatment of drug addiction: "A difficult and most ungracious task"' *Harm Reduction Journal* (2011), 8:32.